40 DAYS TO
BETTER LIVING

WEIGHT MANAGEMENT

BARBOUR
PUBLISHING

ISBN 978-1-61626-267-9

Published by Barbour Publishing, Inc., P.O. Box 719, Uhrichsville, Ohio 44683
www.barbourbooks.com

Our mission is to publish and distribute inspirational products offering exceptional value and biblical encouragement to the masses.

 Member of the
Evangelical Christian
Publishers Association

Printed in the United States of America.

CONTENTS

Welcome
From Dr. Scott Morris
Founder of the Church Health Center

I first came to Memphis in 1986. I had no personal ties to Memphis and did not know anyone here. Having completed theological and medical education, I was determined to begin a health care ministry for the working poor. The next year, the doors of the Church Health Center opened with one doctor— me—and one nurse. We saw twelve patients the first day. Today we handle about 36,000 patient visits a year and 120,000 visits to our Wellness facility. A staff of 250 people shares a ministry of healing and wellness while hundreds more volunteer time and services.

So what sets us apart from other community clinics around the country?

The Church Health Center is fundamentally about the church. We care for our patients without relying on government funds because God calls the church to healing work. Jesus' life was about healing the whole person—body and spirit—and the church is Jesus in the world. His message is our message. His ministry is our ministry. Local congregations embrace this calling and help make our work possible.

More than two decades of caring for the working uninsured makes one thing plain:

> Jesus' life was about healing the whole person— body and spirit.

health care needs to change. In the years that the Church Health Center has cared for people in Memphis, we've seen that two-thirds of our patients seek treatment for illness that healthier living can prevent or control. We realize that if we want to make a lasting difference in our patients' lives, the most effective strategy is encouraging overall wellness in body and spirit. At a fundamental level, we must transform what the words "well" and "health" mean in the minds of most people.

To do that, we developed the Model for Healthy Living. Living healthy lives doesn't just mean that you see the doctor regularly. Rather, healthy living means that all aspects of your life are in balance. Your faith, work, nutrition, movement, family and friends, emotions, and medical health all contribute to a life filled with more joy, more love, and more connection to God.

How to Use This Book

This book gives you the chance to improve your health in whatever way is needed for managing your weight. For the next forty days, we invite you to be inspired by the real-life people whose lives have been changed by the Church Health Center. Each day gives us a new chance to more effectively manage our weight, so each day we will give you helpful ways that you can make your life a healthier one.

Some days you may choose to focus on just one or two of our "tips": Faith Life, Medical, Movement, Work, Emotional, Family and Friends, or Nutrition. Some days you may want to try all of them. The important thing is to remember that God calls us to an abundant life, and we can always make changes to strive for better health as it relates to our weight.

Forty days and numerous ways to live a healthy life—come and join us on the journey!

Growing up on a farm, Andrew was always thin.

He enjoyed the outdoors and spent most of his time walking the acres of the farm. He was so thin, however, that his family thought there was something wrong with him. They were all very large, and his thinness set him apart. Andrew says he wasn't accepted by his family because of his size.

When he left the farm and went away to college, Andrew stopped walking almost entirely. He ate a lot of cafeteria food, stopped exercising, and steadily gained more and more weight. After college, Andrew found that his family now considered him too heavy instead of too thin. He became depressed and angry about his family's continual rejection based on his size.

As Andrew's depression deepened, he had a tough time finding work, and soon he started having financial problems. He found himself without a car and started walking again—this time out of necessity. As he walked, he started losing weight, his mood elevated, and he remembered all those times on the farm that he so enjoyed. Andrew realized that he needed to take a long, hard look at his perceptions of his body and came to the Church Health Center for support. With a few years of diligent work, Andrew now maintains a healthy, balanced weight and is working to overcome his problems with his family.

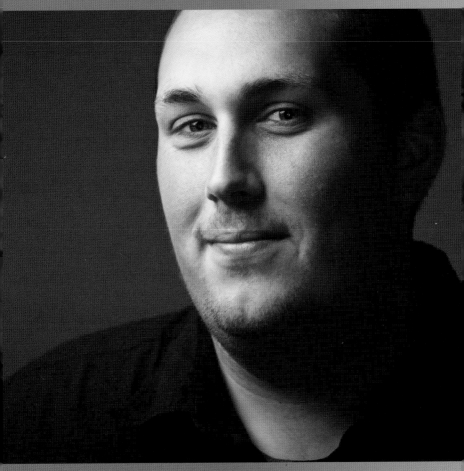

Andrew says he wasn't accepted by his family because of his size.

Morning Reflection

Welcome! Today is the first day of your weight-management journey. Whether you want to lose, gain, or maintain weight, this trek is about finding the right balance for a healthy and wellness-oriented lifestyle. As we begin this journey, we must remember that steps along the way—especially first steps—can be both exhilarating and intimidating. Achieving a healthy weight is not just about dieting. The journey to wellness is about transforming your life—inside and out. So today we will consider what this journey means to us.

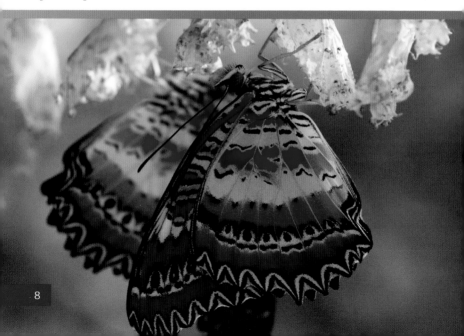

»Faith Life

If you do not already have a journal, start one today. This is a place where you can record faith and emotional reflections as well as the progress that you will make on your journey.

»Medical

Part of beginning is knowing where you are when you start. Do you have any medical concerns? Today make a list of those concerns. Include major concerns, like chronic conditions, as well as smaller issues, like acne or skin conditions.

»Movement

Today, to discover your starting point, go for a walk. Walk for as long as you can without exhausting yourself. Make a note of how long you were able to walk.

{ Achieving a healthy weight is not just about dieting. }

»Work

Work means different things to different people. Sometimes it can mean a job, and sometimes it means volunteering, raising children, or gardening. Today make a list of where you work and what you like about your work.

»Emotional

You can use this book to start a journal. You can also use your computer, a separate journal, or loose-leaf paper. But keeping a journal is very important to the process, so today (if you have not already started one) begin writing in a journal.

»Family and Friends

Personal relationships, both family and friends, are crucial to overall wellness. They provide support and laughter and engagement. Make a list of the personal relationships you can depend on.

»Nutrition

An excellent way to keep track of your nutritional habits (even those you may not be aware of) is to keep a food journal. Today start keeping a log of what and how much you eat.

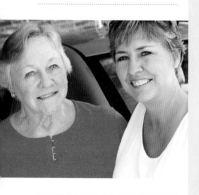

Evening Wrap-Up

Beginnings are a part of life, no matter where we might be on the journey. Today marks a new beginning and a first step on a journey toward weight management and wellness. And as we set out on this journey, we can be certain that God walks with us. After all, the first verse in Genesis tells us about the beginning that God has already experienced. "The earth was formless and empty. . . ." As we take our first steps on this journey, we may feel like the road ahead is formless and empty, but God is with us and can give us the courage and encouragement we need.

In the beginning God created the heavens and the earth. Now the earth was formless and empty, darkness was over the surface of the deep, and the Spirit of God was hovering over the waters.

GENESIS 1:1–2

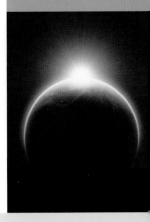

Loving God, give me strength today and walk with me as I set out on this journey to weight management and wellness. In Your holy name, Amen.

Morning Reflection

In our communities and in our current culture, flesh often gets a bad rap. We constantly critique ourselves, thinking that we have too much or too little. We might berate ourselves for "giving in" to the temptations of "the flesh." But part of this journey will be realizing that we are created *in the flesh*. A portion of our transformation must be learning to love the fleshy bodies that we are given and appreciating the fleshy lives that we live.

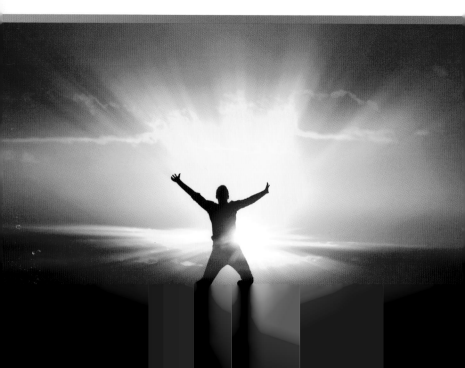

»Faith Life

Our faith lives often ignore "flesh" or treat "flesh" as if it were always negative. Today write five ways that your body is important to your faith life. For example, do you use your hands to pray? Do you sing in church?

....

....

....

....

....

....

....

....

{
Part of this journey will be realizing that we are created *in the flesh*.
}

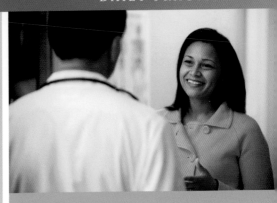

»Medical

When was the last time you had a physical with a doctor? If it has been more than a year, call your doctor today to set up an appointment.

....

....

....

»Movement

Movement is all about the flesh. Today try doing some light stretching after a short walk. Stretch your arms across your chest, reach down to your toes, stretch your back, and roll your neck. Feel the way your body moves.

....

....

....

....

13

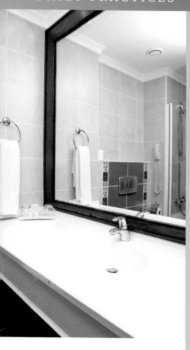

» Work

What do you like about your work? What do you dislike? Take five minutes and write some things that you like and dislike about your work. (Remember, work can be your job/career, but can also be volunteering, parenting, etc.)

» Emotional

We can get very emotional about our flesh. So today stand in front of a mirror (full length, if you have it). Then, in your journal, write down five things that you like about your body.

» Family and Friends

Do you eat family dinners? Family dinners are a wonderful way to spend time with your family, catching up and talking. They are also wonderful times to try new recipes. Take time today to think of a good evening for a family dinner in the next week.

» Nutrition

Do you have a standard grocery list each week? Today make a list of your usual grocery list. Include drinks, snacks, and meals on your list.

Evening Wrap-Up

As we begin our weight-management journey, we can begin

to appreciate that God chose to live on Earth *in the flesh.* Because God chose to become flesh, we can rest in the assurance that flesh is good. Our flesh is a gift—one that, in our current culture, we spend a lot of time trying to give back. So on this journey, we will try to learn how to love and value our flesh.

In the beginning was the Word, and the Word was with God, and the Word was God. He was with God in the beginning. . . . In him was life, and that life was the light of all mankind. The light shines in the darkness, and the darkness has not overcome it. . . . The Word became flesh and made his dwelling among us. We have seen his glory, the glory of the one and only Son, who came from the Father, full of grace and truth.

JOHN 1:1–2, 4–5, 14

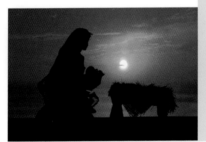

Loving God, help me to care for my body the way that You care for me. In Your holy name, Amen.

Morning Reflection

We all set out on the journey toward wellness for different reasons. Sometimes it is as simple as getting ready for "bathing suit season," but if we want to make lasting changes, we need to identify our larger purpose on the journey. Maybe we want to be healthy so we can set a good example for our children or so we can go for a run comfortably. Managing weight is a lifelong journey, and understanding our larger purpose on the journey can help give us direction.

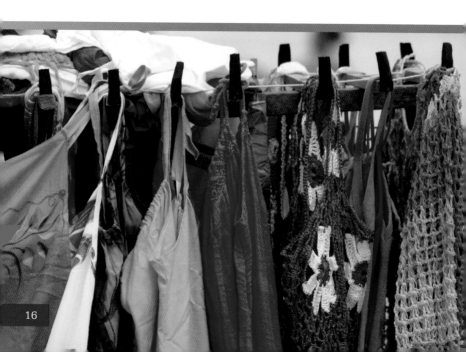

» Faith Life

Our faith can be a guiding force in our lives. Today spend ten minutes writing in your journal about how your faith life has shaped your purpose. Has your faith life influenced your decision to set out on this journey toward wellness?

» Medical

Do you have a family history of medical issues? (Examples include hypertension, heart disease, and diabetes.) Perhaps your family history is a part of the reason you started this journey. Make a list of your family medical history and discuss it with your doctor the next time you see him or her.

» Movement

Go for a walk today, as far as you can go. Take a break when you need it, and walk a little longer. As you walk, think about how you feel now and how you would like to feel two weeks from now, six weeks from now.

» Work

Return to the list you made yesterday of things you like and dislike about your work. What would you like to change about your work? What do you have the power and authority to change in your work?

» Emotional

Why did you decide to begin the journey toward wellness? Take ten minutes today and write your purpose. Include your "big picture" understanding.

» Family and Friends

Family and friends often provide a good deal of motivation as well as support. Today have a conversation with a friend or family member about your purpose. This way, when you experience setbacks, you will have someone who can help to remind you of your purpose.

» Nutrition

What are the most important things to you about your food? Calorie count? Taste? Cost? Make a list of the five most important qualities of your food. In the weeks to come, we will try to learn healthy ways to have food that still meets the qualities that you value most.

Evening Wrap-Up:

*Forgetting what
is behind and
straining toward
what is ahead,
I press on toward
the goal to win
the prize for which
God has called
me heavenward in
Christ Jesus.*

PHILIPPIANS
3:13–14

Finding our larger purpose on the journey means keeping the bigger picture in view. This broader view can help us get back on track when we have setbacks. In his letter to the Philippians, Paul writes about "straining toward what is ahead." Sure, swimsuit season is ahead, but so is life. The bigger picture in the journey toward weight management and wellness is life. What lies ahead of us is life, and life in abundance, which God has promised each of us who know Him. So as we press on toward the goal, we can rest assured that God walks the journey with us.

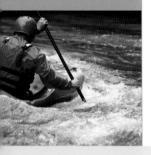

God of wisdom, help me to keep the bigger picture in view.
Thank You for continuing to walk with me on this journey toward wellness.
In Your holy name, Amen.

Morning Reflection

Just like having a long-term vision for your journey is important, so is having short-term goals to function like mile markers on your journey. These short-term goals need to be realistic and action oriented, and can be very valuable in giving encouragement as the journey progresses. So today we will turn our focus to setting doable and realistic goals that can be achieved in the next six weeks.

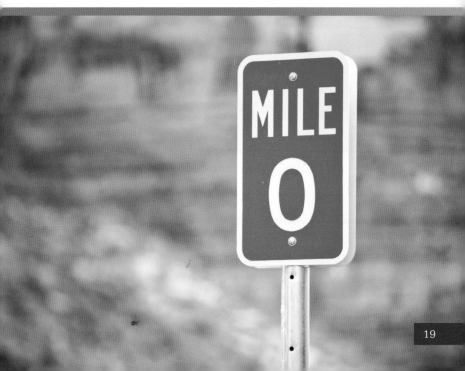

»Medical

Before you begin any kind of serious exercise program, make sure that you speak to your doctor. Know with as much certainty as possible what your limits are before you begin.

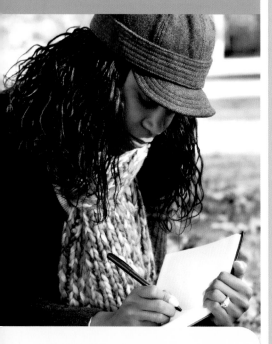

»Faith Life

Take ten minutes today and write ten words that describe your faith life. Then write ten words that you would like to describe your faith life. Try to be honest. Remember, no one will see the list except for you.

»Movement

Write down five movement goals to accomplish in the next six weeks. If you are not a runner, remember that "run a marathon" is probably not a reasonable goal for the next six weeks. However, "walk a mile" might be a more reasonable goal. Keep in mind your current level of fitness and go from there.

{ Today we will spend some time considering what our expectations are of ourselves and of God. }

»Work

Make a list of five of your wellness goals and take them with you to your workplace. This will help to remind you what you are trying to accomplish during the day. Having the goals in plain sight may also inspire you to be creative in achieving those goals.

»Emotional

For many of us, the only time we set goals is around New Year's. Today take five minutes and write about how setting goals makes you feel. Do you feel excited? Intimidated?

»Family and Friends

Are you embarking on this journey on your own or with a friend or some family members? Having a companion who is going through the same journey can be very helpful. Think today about a friend or family member whom you might reach out to for support.

»Nutrition

What would you like to change about your nutritional habits? Eat less fat? More vegetables? Better portion sizes? Write down five nutritional goals for the next six weeks.

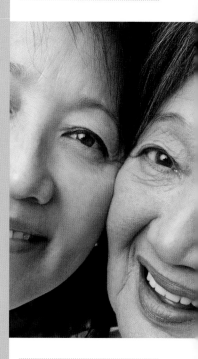

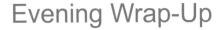

Evening Wrap-Up

*"Listen to me,
you descendants of
Jacob, all the remnant
of the people of Israel,
you whom I have upheld
since your birth. . .
Even to your old age
and gray hairs I am he,
I am he who will sustain
you. I have made you
and I will carry you;
I will sustain you and
I will rescue you."*

ISAIAH 46:3–4

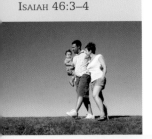

Even on day four of this journey,

it can be easy to become intimidated. Although we set reasonable and practical goals, the journey might seem overwhelming and even impossible at times. But as we set out on the journey, we can know that God cares for us and walks with us. In this passage from Isaiah, God tells us, "I have made you and I will carry you." What greater assurance do we need that God is with us?

Loving God, I know that You have carried me since my birth. Be with me as I walk this journey toward wellness. In Your holy name, Amen.

Morning Reflection

Whether we want to admit it or not, we all come to this journey with expectations of what the coming weeks will look like. Some of our expectations are reasonable, while some may be setting us up for disappointment. Unrealistic expectations can (and do!) shape our overall experience, making us feel like giving up if the journey does not live up to those expectations. So today we will take some time and explore what our expectations are for the road ahead.

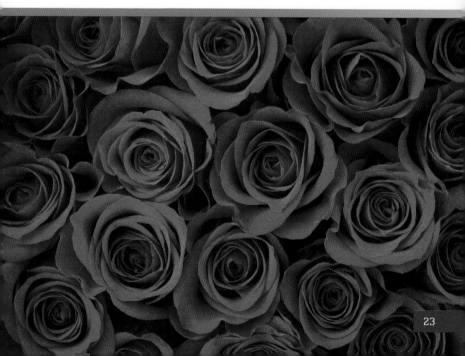

» Faith Life

We all have expectations as a part of our faith lives, including expectations of God. Today take five minutes and write about your expectations of God.

» Medical

If you do not know how to find your pulse, today is the day to learn! Use your index and middle fingers to feel your pulse at your wrist. Count the beats that you feel for 15 seconds and multiply the number by four. That is your resting heart rate.

» Movement

Spend ten minutes stretching today. Can you stretch a bit farther than you could a couple of days ago? What are your expectations for a few days from now?

» Work

Do you expect that your work life will change at all on this journey? If so, how? If not, why not? Take five minutes and write in your journal about how your work life can be a part of your wellness journey.

» Emotional

Our expectations can seriously impact our emotional well-being. Take five minutes and write in your journal about what your expectations are for this journey to weight management and wellness. Try to be honest. Are there any that you know are probably unrealistic?

» Family and Friends

Sometimes we feel that our family and friends have particular expectations of us, and that can add to the stress that we are already feeling. Talk to a friend or family member today about your journey and what your expectations are.

» Nutrition

What kinds of food do you like to eat? Take five minutes and make a list of your favorite foods. Are they healthy foods? Comfort foods? As this journey progresses, you may be able to modify your favorite foods with healthier versions.

Evening Wrap-Up

This journey, just like every excursion, will be full of ups and downs. It will be full of mountains and molehills, good days and bad. If we expect every day to be a complete success, then we are likely to feel let down or discouraged. As we continue on this journey, remember that God is with us through all our highs and lows. The author of Ecclesiastes reminds us that there are good times and bad, and that we can celebrate the good times, even while being comforted in the bad times.

When times are good, be happy; but when times are bad, consider this: God has made the one as well as the other.

ECCLESIASTES 7:14

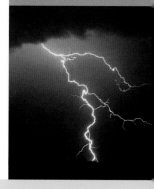

God of the journey, thank You for making all days, good and bad. Help me today and on the days ahead to remember that You have made all of my days. In Your holy name, Amen.

Morning Reflection

Setbacks are a part of life. As we move forward, we will experience obstacles. But with setbacks come opportunities to learn and grow. They give us the chance to better understand ourselves and our limitations. But setbacks can also open our eyes to strengths and abilities that we did not realize we had. So as we move forward on this journey, we can view setbacks as opportunities, rather than as deal breakers.

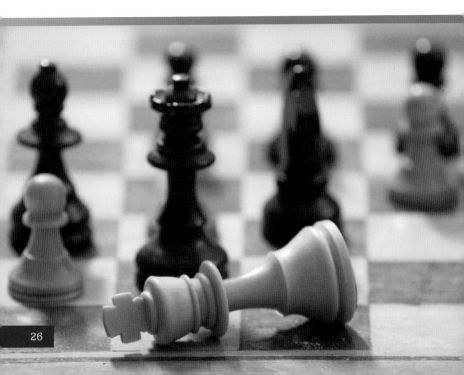

»Faith Life

Most of us have had both significant and minor setbacks in faith at some point in our lives. Take five minutes today and write about a time when you stumbled in your faith life. How did you manage to move forward? What did you learn from the experience?

....

....

....

....

....

....

....

{ Making true progress involves a lot of moving forward and then dealing with setbacks. }

»Medical

While medical setbacks can be devastating, they need not be the end of the world. If you have had a medical setback, talk to your doctor about developing a strategy to overcome it.

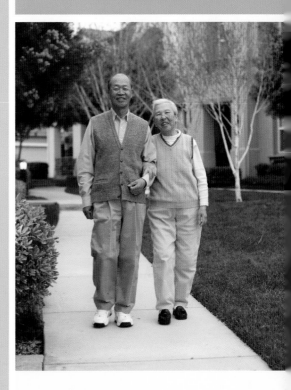

»Movement

Spend ten minutes walking around your house (or walk around your neighborhood if you feel comfortable) taking two steps forward and one step backward. Notice that you still move forward. And walking backward exercises different muscles than walking forward.

27

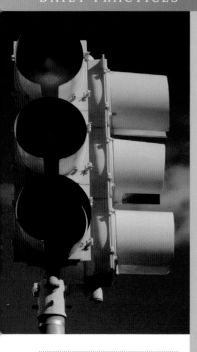

» Work
How do setbacks affect your attitude about work? Do you become less engaged in work? Or do you throw yourself into the job? Think about how your experience at work, either positive or negative, can cause setbacks at home.

» Emotional
Setbacks are perhaps the most devastating for our emotional health, because we can convince ourselves that moving forward after we slip is impossible. Today think of a strategy to deal with emotional setbacks. (For example, decide to take a day off, go for a walk, and start again the next day.)

» Family and Friends
Personal relationships are very important in the event of a setback, because they can offer you encouragement and perspective that you may not have for yourself. Identify two people in your life who are particularly gifted in offering you encouragement when you need it.

» Nutrition
Nutritional setbacks happen. We give in to the temptation of a doughnut or eat too much at a friend's birthday dinner. The temptation is to starve ourselves the day after to "make up" for the setback. Instead, just get back on track eating a healthy and reasonable diet.

Evening Wrap-Up

As we travel the journey to wellness, we will likely find that the path is not always straight, even, or particularly easy to walk. There will be times when the road gets more difficult. There may even be times when we simply need to sit and rest. However, this does not mean that the journey ends each time we have a setback. Paul reminds us that what we perceive as foolishness can be wisdom in God's sight. The stumbling blocks on our journey can be sources of great wisdom and growth if we allow them to be.

Do not deceive yourselves. If any of you think you are wise by the standards of this age, you should become "fools" so that you may become wise. For the wisdom of this world is foolishness in God's sight.

1 CORINTHIANS 3:18–19

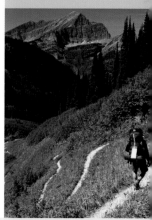

Loving God, grant me the vision to see growth in my setbacks on this journey. In Your holy name, Amen.

Morning Reflection

Congratulations! You've made it to the end of week one! You've taken your first steps on the journey and can now look forward to the weeks to come. But before you dive into the next steps, pause, reflect on the week behind you, and celebrate the distance you've traveled already. As we continue on, it is important to occasionally pause, take stock, and yes, celebrate. Today we will turn our focus to the celebration at week's end.

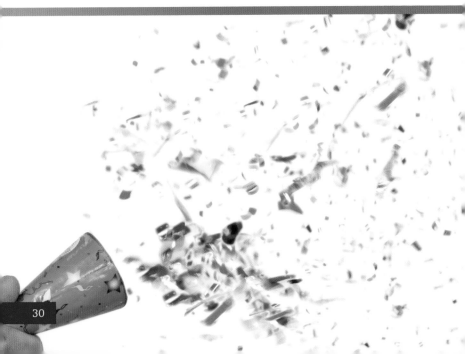

»Faith Life

Faith is an important part of wellness, but wellness is also important to faith. Keep in mind that God entered this world as a person with a body. Go for a walk today, and pray as you walk for God to be present in your body as well as your spirit.

»Medical

Do you remember how to check your pulse? Try again today to calculate your resting heart rate. Knowing your numbers will help you track your improvement throughout the next five weeks.

»Movement

Spend ten minutes in an activity that gets your heart rate up. Go for a walk, or do some jumping jacks. Try to make it an activity that you enjoy doing.

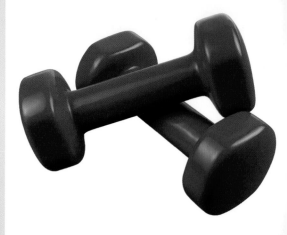

{ Congratulations! You have reached the end of the first week. }

»Work

Take some small (two- to five-pound) hand weights to work to keep at your desk. If you have a minute or two, do a few sets of simple bicep curls or shoulder presses to work your upper body a bit.

»Emotional

Write in your journal how you are feeling about the journey thus far. Are you excited? Tired? Encouraged? What does the "horizon" look like for you?

»Family and Friends

Have a small celebration with your family or some friends for getting through your first week. Do something that you enjoy doing with your family.

»Nutrition

Make a grocery list that looks forward. Include plenty of whole grains, fresh vegetables and fruits, and limit the prepared and processed foods.

Evening Wrap-Up

Many of us have become used to viewing steps on the journey as simple events that deserve little celebration, if any. But the truth is that celebration is a part of the journey. Also, as we travel this journey, remember that God travels and celebrates with us. In this passage from Isaiah we are told, "Your heart will throb and swell with joy." Joy and celebration are as much a part of this journey as portion control.

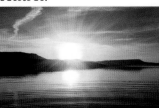

"Arise, shine, for your light has come, and the glory of the LORD rises upon you. See, darkness covers the earth and thick darkness is over the peoples, but the LORD rises upon you and his glory appears over you. Nations will come to your light, and kings to the brightness of your dawn. . . . Then you will look and be radiant, your heart will throb and swell with joy."

ISAIAH 60:1–3, 5

Joyous God, help me today to celebrate the steps that I have taken on this journey. In Your holy name, Amen.

Nella suffered from severe obesity her entire life. She found support at Church Health Center Wellness and started losing weight—ten, twenty, then forty pounds—but she was getting very impatient to meet her goal of losing over a hundred pounds. As her frustration grew, Nella began pushing herself too hard. She was weighing herself several times a day, exercising to sheer exhaustion, and crying every time she didn't have a significant loss of weight.

One day Nella was exercising with her exercise specialist, Frank, and commented to him that she felt the fifty-three pounds she had lost were a waste. She just couldn't feel good about it because it wasn't enough, and she felt like she had so far to go. She was losing her motivation because she still "felt fat."

Frank thought a moment and then remembered that Nella had brought her granddaughter Kendra to exercise with her. Frank asked Kendra to step on a scale, and she weighed right at fifty pounds. Then Frank asked Nella to pick up her grandchild and try to carry her around for a while, doing her exercises and going on about her day. Nella tried for a few moments but couldn't keep holding Kendra—she was too heavy.

When Nella put her granddaughter down, she said that she understood how far she had come in her weight management. She was relieved that her body was carrying a lighter load, but more importantly, she was grateful for the constant care that God provides—even when the results were too subtle for her to notice immediately.

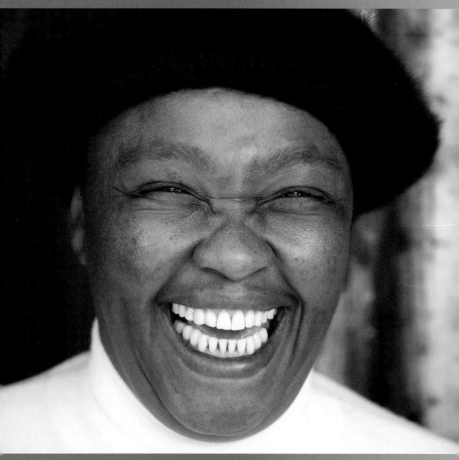

She was relieved that her body was carrying a lighter load, but more importantly, she was grateful for the constant care that God provides—even when the results were too subtle for her to notice immediately.

Weight Management

Morning Reflection

We all have habits—both good and bad. We have them in all aspects of our lives, and this journey is largely about identifying and changing some of those habits. As we all know, changing habits is tricky, largely because they are behaviors that have become automatic. We step into them without even thinking! Now we'll try to learn how to think about our habits so we're not always controlled by them.

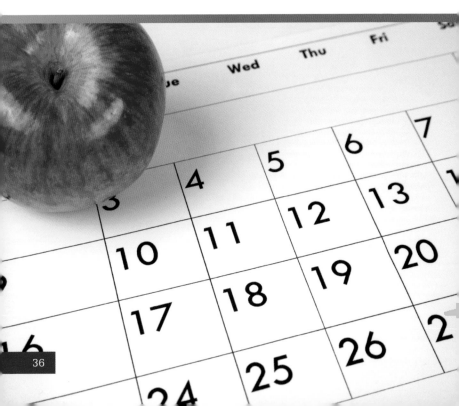

»Faith Life

Today take five minutes and make a list of some of your faith habits. Do you pray at a regular time? Do you read the Bible at night? Try to set up a regular time to pray if you do not already have one.

{ Changing habits is tricky. }

»Medical

Do you have a list of all your medications and where they can be found? Make a list (either by hand or on a computer) and put it on your refrigerator. That way, if you ever have an emergency, your list of medications is readily available.

1
2
3

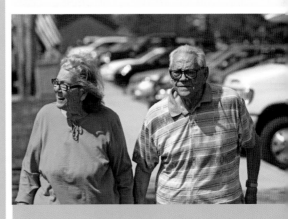

»Movement

How much movement and exercise do you get on an average day? Today try to keep track of how often you move. For example, do you walk from the parking lot to the door? How far? Add up all your small movements today.

»Work

What are your habits when you get home from work? Do you eat? Clean? Watch television? Pay attention today to the small things you do. Write down your actions in fifteen-minute increments. You may be surprised!

»Emotional

We often have emotional ups and downs over the course of the day. Today pay special attention to when you feel those highs and lows. How do you feel in the morning? After lunch? In the evening? Write down in your journal when you have your highs and lows.

»Family and Friends

Do you have things that you often do with your family and friends? What are they? Spend a few minutes writing a list of the things that you like to do with the people in your life.

»Nutrition

Don't drink your calories! Substitute water for sweetened drinks such as sweetened iced tea or soda. If you want something fizzy, try drinking seltzer water.

Evening Wrap-Up

Our habits are so deeply ingrained

that we can easily catch ourselves falling into behaviors without even knowing it. This is the very thing that can make altering our behavior a discouraging, messy process. But Paul assures us that we can work to change our habits, and that God will be with us as we do. He tells us to "put on the full armor of God." We can clothe ourselves with the encouragement that God offers us as we continue on our wellness journey.

Take up the shield of faith. . . . Take the helmet of salvation and the sword of the Spirit, which is the word of God. And pray in the Spirit on all occasions with all kinds of prayers and requests. With this in mind, be alert and always keep on praying for all the Lord's people.

EPHESIANS
6:16–18

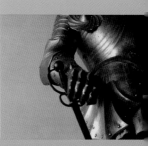

Loving God, thank You for walking on this journey with me. Grant me encouragement as I work to change my habits. In Your holy name, Amen.

Morning Reflection

Every day, even as we get out of bed in the morning, we face stress. We face good stress and bad stress, and we need to learn how to differentiate between good stress and bad. Moreover, we need to learn how to cope with the bad stress so we don't become overwhelmed. It's when we become overwhelmed that we resort to the old and comfortable (and often unhealthy) behaviors. Today we will focus on ways to manage our stress.

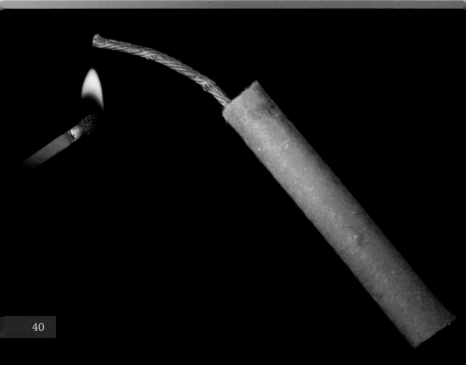

»Faith Life

Often as a part of our faith life, we neglect to sit quietly and listen or meditate. Today spend five minutes sitting quietly and breathing. Try to quiet your inner voice and just listen.

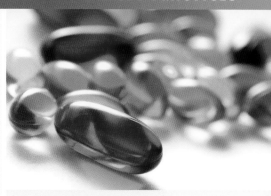

»Medical

In addition to having a list of your medications posted on your refrigerator, make sure that a close relative or friend has a list of your medications and recommended dosages.

{ Triggers are emotions or events that "turn on" our habits. }

»Movement

Often our response to stress might be to eat or to sit in front of the television. Today if you feel stress, try to go for a walk or do some jumping jacks to give yourself some relief.

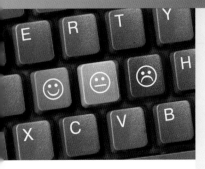

» Work

How do you respond to stress at work?
If you feel stress on the job today, try taking a short walk or squeeze a stress ball. Taking some time away from your work and doing something entirely different can help you to relax and breathe.

» Emotional

When you feel stress, how do you deal with it? Take five minutes today and imagine a stressful situation that you had recently. Write about how you dealt with that stress.

» Family and Friends

Sometimes being with family stresses us out. In particular, having the responsibility that often comes with family can add to our stress. Today make sure that you take some time (even if it's only a couple of minutes) to have time to yourself when you need it.

» Nutrition

Meal planning can also be stressful at times. To make meal planning less stressful, try planning out meals in advance and preparing as much as you can on the weekend. That way you'll be less tempted to resort to fast food because you don't know what to have for dinner.

Evening Wrap-Up

On our weight-management journey, stress will always play a large factor. We hear a good deal about how we, as a culture, are "stressed out." We often cope with this stress in unhealthy ways, such as habitually eating and drinking or even withdrawing from friends and family. In the letter to the Hebrews, the author reminds us that we can continue to run the race set before us and not lose heart.

Therefore, since we are surrounded by such a great cloud of witnesses, let us throw off everything that hinders and the sin that so easily entangles. And let us run with perseverance the race marked out for us, fixing our eyes on Jesus, the pioneer and perfecter of faith. . . so that you will not grow weary and lose heart.

HEBREWS 12:1–3

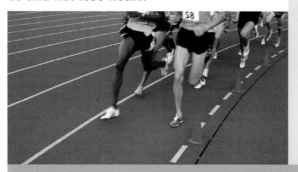

Merciful Lord, help me today when I become overwhelmed to breathe and to not grow weary. In Your holy name, Amen.

Morning Reflection

As we nurture our wellness, we will find areas where we need to make room—clean house, both literally and figuratively—so we can continue to grow. Sometimes we need to take time to clean out our pantries and our refrigerators. Sometimes we also need to take the time to clean out our spirits and our bodies to make room for healthier meals and behaviors. Today we will focus on ways to make room for wellness on our weight-management journey.

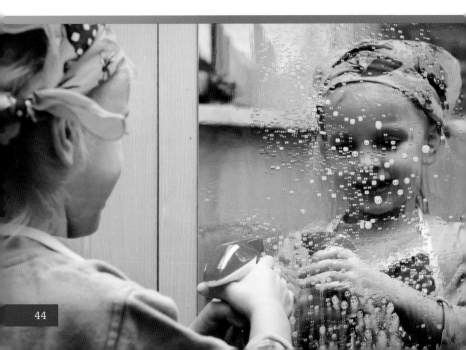

» Faith Life

Yesterday you spent time meditating and listening. Today spend ten minutes sitting quietly again. Try to quiet your mind, clear out the clutter—the stress and anxiety. Breathe and hear God.

» Medical

When was the last time you cleaned out your medicine cabinet? Lots of accidents can be avoided by disposing of expired and old medication. Today take inventory of your medicine cabinet and throw out anything expired or unusable.

» Movement

Is a messy house or room keeping you from exercising or eating properly? Spend a half hour today decluttering one area of your house. When you're finished, you might feel better and less overwhelmed.

» Work

Clear out a space at your work (in your desk or somewhere convenient) where you can keep some healthy snacks on hand. When you take a break, instead of going to a vending machine, enjoy a healthy snack and a short walk.

» Emotional

Set aside some time today to take a warm bath. Even spending a few minutes soaking in a tub can help to relax your muscles. Do some deep breathing as you soak.

» Family and Friends

Recruit some of your family and friends to help you clean out your kitchen. Throw out expired foods, as well as processed foods with a high sugar or fat content.

» Nutrition

Move the unhealthy snacks, such as potato chips or cookies, out of reach and out of sight. Set them on a high shelf in the pantry or throw them out entirely. Move healthy snacks, such as fresh vegetables or fruits, into places where you can see them and grab them easily.

Evening Wrap-Up

Have you heard the expression "clearing the brush"? Clearing the brush means getting rid of the grass and scrub so that other plants can grow. It's about making room for new growth. On this road to wellness, we need to occasionally take the time to clear space so we can see the task ahead of us. Even in this passage from Proverbs, we are reminded that the hay must be removed before new growth appears.

When the hay is removed and new growth appears and the grass from the hills is gathered in, the lambs will provide you with clothing, and the goats with the price of a field. You will have plenty of goats' milk to feed your family and to nourish your female servants.

PROVERBS 27:25–27

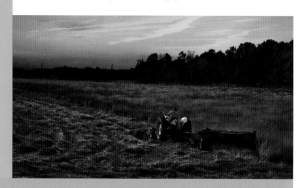

Loving God, help me today as I clear away the hay to make room for new growth. In Your holy name, Amen.

Morning Reflection

When we talk about "triggers," we mean external factors that "trigger" behaviors in us, sometimes without our even noticing. For example, have you ever found yourself ordering popcorn at the movies, even when you're not hungry? Each day is full of these triggers and the behaviors that we can fall into automatically. Today we will focus on how to recognize our triggers and the behaviors that go with them. In recognizing them, we can gain some power over them and change our behavior.

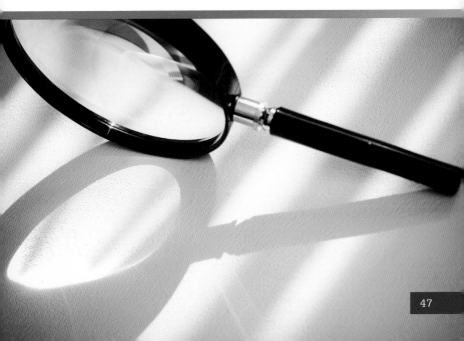

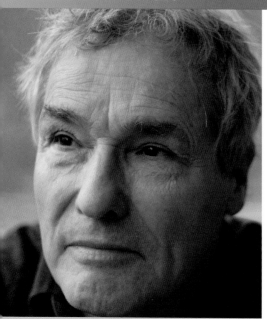

»Faith Life

Today take five minutes to pray in a way that you have never prayed before. Try writing or even singing a prayer. Sometimes purposefully breaking out of a pattern can help us recognize patterns—even where we might not have noticed them before.

»Movement

Many of us eat when we feel bored or overwhelmed. Today if you feel bored (but are not actually hungry), instead of snacking, try doing some simple stretches, such as neck rolls and arm crosses.

»Medical

Some vitamins and supplements can keep us healthy rather than trying to fix what is wrong. Ask your doctor about some vitamin supplements that can potentially improve your health.

> Our overall wellness is dependent on our attitude toward wellness.

»Work

What are your triggers at work? Do you always take a coffee break at a certain time? Eat lunch from the vending machine? Try replacing your coffee with herbal tea and bringing a lunch from home.

»Emotional

What do you do when you feel happy? When you feel sad? Bored? Take five minutes and write in your journal, thinking about how you usually behave when faced with these emotions.

»Family and Friends

Family can be one of the biggest triggers of all, because when families get together, we have long-standing patterns of behavior, emotion—and especially eating! If your family is gathering today, try to focus on the fellowship rather than the food.

»Nutrition

If you do feel like snacking today, try some unsalted nuts or dried fruits instead of sugary or salty snacks like cookies and chips.

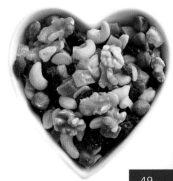

49

As the deer pants for streams of water, so my soul pants for you, my God. My soul thirsts for God, for the living God. When can I go and meet with God? . . . These things I remember as I pour out my soul: how I used to go to the house of God under the protection of the Mighty One with shouts of joy and praise among the festive throng.

PSALM 42:1–2, 4

Evening Wrap-Up

Every day we encounter and respond to dozens of triggers.

Stress, sadness, nervousness—even happiness—can initiate behaviors in us that we may not understand or even see. But the psalmist assures us that there is always a deeper, stronger longing, and that is the longing of our soul for God. Because we are built with that longing, we can know that God is always with us as we walk this path toward wellness.

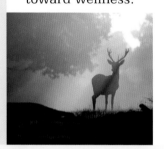

God, in every moment of life, as I continue on this journey, give me courage to face my triggers and to know that I can respond differently. In Your holy name, Amen.

Morning Reflection

As we learn more about wellness, we will be altering and shaping not just our bodies, but the way we see and understand our entire person. Our culture has a tendency to see each individual as a series of parts—legs, eyes, toes, voices. But that is not how we are created. We are created as whole selves—complete and good. Today we will turn our focus toward appreciating the wholeness we were created with.

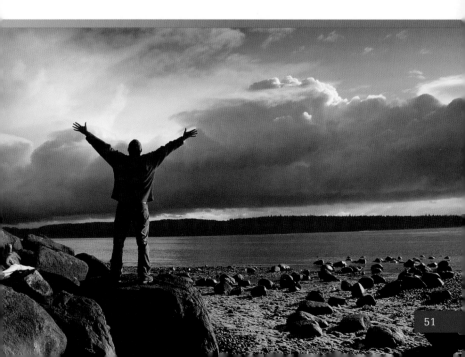

» Faith Life

When you pray today, wiggle your fingers and your toes. Stand up and sit down. Jump up and down. Breathe in and out. Think about how our whole bodies can pray.

» Medical

In addition to prescription medication, do you take over-the-counter medication and/or vitamins? Be certain to include those on your list of medications for the refrigerator and emergency contacts.

» Movement

Put on some music. Spend five minutes today dancing to the music in whatever way you can dance. Move your whole body as much as you can. Move your head, your back, your fingers, your toes. Feel your entire body working together.

» Work

Most of us work using one aspect of our personality more than other parts. Today try to take five minutes at work and use another aspect of your body or personality. If you sit at a computer all day, go for a short walk. If you're on the phone, take a moment to stretch, and if you stand all day, find a quiet place to sit.

» Emotional

Sometimes we can feel pulled in seventeen different directions at the same time. To pull yourself together and feel whole, take a shower, let yourself relax, and breathe before getting back to your life.

» Family and Friends

Healthy relationships are very important to wellness and wholeness. Today spend some time enjoying the company of your family and friends. Forget about the "shoulds"—just enjoy socializing and having fun!

» Nutrition

Just as there are many parts to a person, balanced nutrition includes nutrients from a variety of foods. Make sure when you prepare meals that you include fruits and vegetables, lean protein, and whole-grain carbohydrates.

Evening Wrap-Up

How many times have we heard this? *We are created in God's image.*

And yet, how often do we look in the mirror and pick apart the image looking back at us? When we pick at ourselves, we are not seeing our entire persons. Instead, we see stomachs or noses or hair. But we are created whole—body and spirit—and God knows us whole—body and spirit. Keep in mind that God has created each of us whole.

Then God said, "Let us make man in our image, in our likeness, so that they may rule over the fish in the sea and the birds in the sky, over the livestock and all the wild animals, and over all the creatures that move along the ground." So God created mankind in his own image, in the image of God he created them; male and female he created them.

GENESIS 1:26–27

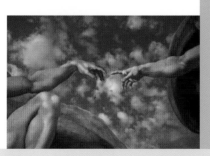

Creator God, I know that I am created whole. I pray today that You would give me eyes to see the wholeness in myself. In Your holy name, Amen.

Morning Reflection

Our journey to wellness will sometimes be smooth and sometimes be rough. But how we navigate the rough patches of the journey depends largely on our attitudes as the journey progresses. It is inevitable that we will occasionally feel discouraged when things don't go as we had planned. To feel discouraged is only human. But it can be entirely too easy to stop when we feel discouraged. Instead, to move forward on the journey and to grow, we need to find ways to continue on the journey, even after discouragement.

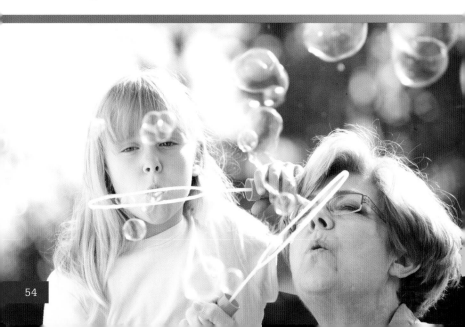

»Faith Life

Take five minutes today and meditate again. Quiet your thoughts and then focus on the blessings that you have received, such as a body that works, wonderful friends, and good food.

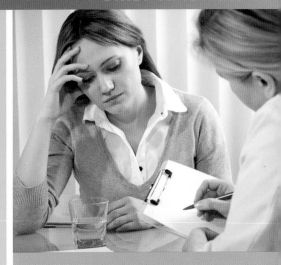

»Medical

Remember that medications can have side effects—some are physical and some are emotional. If you are having emotional side effects (such as depression, anxiety, euphoria) or physical side effects, let your doctor know as soon as possible.

{ The journey to wellness is not always smooth. }

»Movement

Exercise can really lift your mood. If you are feeling negative, try doing thirty jumping jacks, and then stretch your arms and back. Even a small amount of exercise can help you to feel more awake and more positive.

» Work

Having a difficult day at work? Instead of focusing on the negative, think of something fun that you can do when you get home, even if it's simply getting outside to enjoy the fresh air. Write it down in a place where you can see your plans for your evening.

» Emotional

Sleep deprivation can really get in the way of having a good attitude. When we are tired, our bodies and brains do not function well. Try to get a good night's sleep, even if it means leaving something undone in your day. You'll feel better when you wake up!

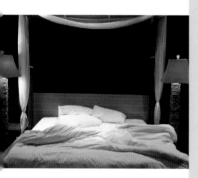

» Family and Friends

Friends are a wonderful resource for dealing with negativity. If you are feeling stressed or overwhelmed, try calling a friend for an emotional pick-me-up. Better yet, suggest that you go for a walk with your friend.

» Nutrition

Cook a delicious and healthy meal for yourself, such as whole-grain pasta or lean meat with steamed vegetables. Eating well reminds us that we can take care of ourselves and can help us maintain a positive attitude.

Evening Wrap-Up

This journey is about many things involving physical health and weight management. But above all, the journey toward wellness is about hope. Just by setting our foot on the path, we admit that we have hope for wellness, change, health, and any number of other things. As we continue on the journey, holding on to hope will help us through the rough moments. In his letter to the Romans, Paul reminds us that God offers hope through the love that He pours into us.

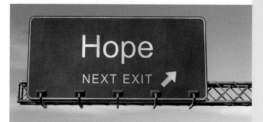

Therefore, since we have been justified through faith, we have peace with God through our Lord Jesus Christ, through whom we have gained access by faith into this grace in which we now stand. And we boast in the hope of the glory of God. Not only so, but we also glory in our sufferings, because we know that suffering produces perseverance; perseverance, character; and character, hope. And hope does not put us to shame, because God's love has been poured out into our hearts through the Holy Spirit, who has been given to us.

Romans 5:1–5

God of love, I know that You love me. I pray that You continue to pour love into me and give me hope for the journey. In Your holy name, Amen.

Morning Reflection

We have arrived at the end of our second week and can now take some time to celebrate and reflect on the days behind us. We have reached another milestone on the journey to wellness. But as we take moments today to celebrate and reflect, let us also take time to be thankful. When we stop to give thanks, we are reminded of how far we have come. Being thankful can balance out the discouragement that we might feel on the journey. Today we will turn our focus to thankfulness.

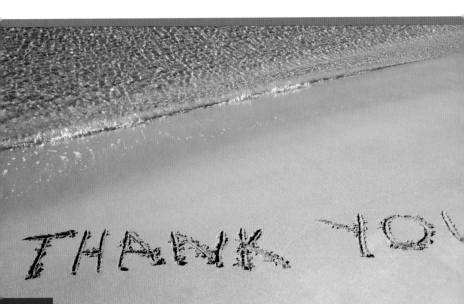

»Faith Life

Thankfulness comes in a variety of forms. Today make a list of everything that you encounter for which you are thankful. At the end of the day, say a prayer, reading the list.

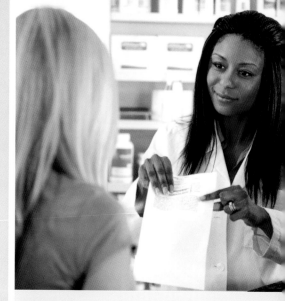

»Medical

Refilling prescriptions can be difficult to remember. If your pharmacy has an automatic refill program, take advantage of it. This way you will never run out of your medication. If you don't need prescription medication, find a way to incorporate daily vitamins into your routine.

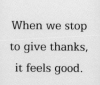

When we stop to give thanks, it feels good.

»Movement

If you are waiting in line today, spend time rising up on your toes and coming back down. This helps to strengthen your calf muscles, which will help build walking endurance.

59

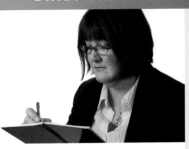

» Work

As you work today, spend some time thinking about the things for which you are thankful. Go for a walk when you are on a break and give thanks for the time you spend walking.

» Emotional

When you are feeling overwhelmed or upset, take five minutes to remember and make a list of the things you are thankful for. This can help you gain perspective.

» Family and Friends

Today take a moment to thank your family and friends for their support. Remember that they are a very important part of your overall wellness.

» Nutrition

If you are a soda drinker and just can't give up the habit, try drinking seltzer water for a carbonated treat. If you want something sweet, try adding a small amount of no-sugar-added fruit juice to the seltzer.

Evening Wrap-Up

We have completed two weeks on the journey! Congratulations! At this point, we can take a moment, pause, and give thanks. As we continue on this journey toward wellness, remembering to be thankful can help us maintain the right perspective. If we feel discouraged, returning to the list of things we are thankful for can anchor us and remind us of the things for which we are blessed.

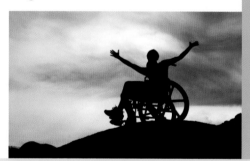

Shout for joy to the Lord, all the earth. Worship the Lord with gladness; come before him with joyful songs. . . . It is he who made us, and we are his; we are his people, the sheep of his pasture. Enter his gates with thanksgiving and his courts with praise; give thanks to him and praise his name. For the Lord is good and his love endures forever; his faithfulness continues through all generations.

PSALM 100

Loving God, I know that You are good and Your love endures forever. For Your love, and for so much more, I am thankful. In Your holy name, Amen.

Geraldine had been a patient at the Church Health Center for many years and had seen almost

every doctor on rotation at the clinic. She was struggling with hypertension, diabetes, and managing her weight, but her troublesome attitude made her a difficult patient to treat, and she never seemed to be happy with the health care she received.

One day she was fed up with what her doctors were telling her and asked to see Dr. Morris, the founder of the center. Dr. Morris came into the room, smiled, and said, "Miss Geraldine, I've looked at your chart and I think you need to go to the Wellness Center. They will help you with your medications and your exercise, and you will feel much better." Geraldine was stunned and began to get agitated. "Why won't you take a look at me? I don't feel well! Don't send me away to some other place!"

Geraldine was angry and determined to prove to Dr. Morris that she was ill and needed medication, not exercise. She went to the Wellness Center and spoke with the health coaches and exercise specialists, who put her on an exercise program. Within just a few weeks, she began to feel better, and after a few more months, she had lost more than twenty pounds and was managing her illnesses better. Now she says, "I set out to prove Dr. Morris wrong. Even though I lost the argument with him, I feel like I won my life back." Then she grins and adds, "But don't tell Dr. Morris he was right!"

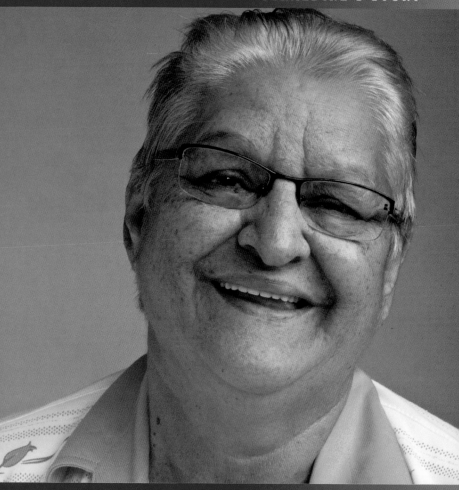

"I set out to prove Dr. Morris wrong. Even though I lost the argument with him, I feel like I won my life back."

Weight Management

Morning Reflection

There is a danger when we set out on our weight-management journey that we will focus entirely on numbers on a scale. But achieving a "goal weight" at any cost can leave us less healthy at the goal weight than we were when we started. So on our journey—the journey with wellness as the ultimate goal—we need to learn how to balance our lifestyle so wellness is the focus.

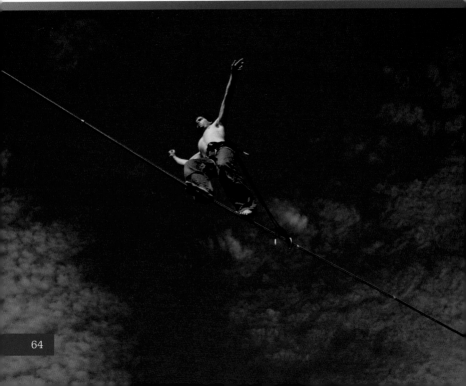

»Faith Life

Read Ecclesiastes 3:1 and take a walk, noticing the careful balance of God's creation. What do you see? What do you hear? What do you smell? Where do you think you fit in the balance?

....

....

....

....

....

....

....

....

....

....

{ We need to learn how to balance our lifestyle. }

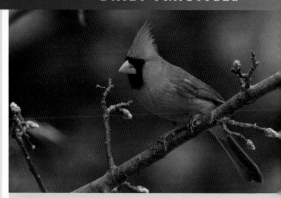

»Medical

Your physical health is about achieving a balance between medications and life-style—between your doctor and you. Today write some questions that you can ask your doctor next time you go in for a check-up.

....

....

....

»Movement

There is no movement without balance! Spend ten minutes today exercising your balance by standing on one leg (one to two minutes on one and then the other, repeating for up to ten minutes). Use a chair or counter-top for support if you need it.

....

....

65

» Work

It can be difficult balancing work and wellness. Today try to add some "wellness balance" to your workday. Take a couple of short walks around the office or just take a couple of moments in the day to breathe and relax.

» Emotional

Emotional balance is sometimes very difficult to maintain, especially with busy schedules. Today find five minutes to balance your business with some quiet time. Spend five minutes sitting and relaxing. Take some deep breaths in and out, close your eyes, and relax.

» Family and Friends

Finding and maintaining your balance is at least partially about knowing when you need to reach out for support. Today try to go for a brisk walk with a friend or family member.

» Nutrition

We've all heard about the importance of a well-balanced diet. Good nutrition is mostly about balance, and balance is about moderation. Portion size can make a huge difference in whether you gain, lose, or maintain weight. Today keep a log of the things that you eat, paying attention to portion size.

Evening Wrap-Up

We live in a world where we are bombarded constantly with

images of celebrities being criticized for carrying a little extra weight or not enough weight. We are offered miracle diets that will give us a "perfect body" in a short amount of time. But all of these things do not create a lasting transformation. Finding wellness, however, means finding balance. In many ways, finding this balance is coming to peace with the balance of God's creation as the author of Ecclesiastes describes it.

All streams flow into the sea, yet the sea is never full. To the place the streams come from, there they return again. . . . The eye never has enough of seeing, nor the ear its fill of hearing. What has been will be again, what has been done will be done again; there is nothing new under the sun.

ECCLESIASTES 1:7–9

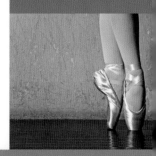

Lord, help me as I continue on this journey to care for myself as You care for all of creation—with balance and love. In Your holy name, Amen.

Morning Reflection

Weight management and wellness are not about extremes. When Geraldine was on her journey to wellness, she bounced around from doctor to doctor trying to hear what she wanted to hear. What she discovered, however, was that wellness was about finding balance, and when she gave herself the space to realize that, her health improved! Sometimes on this journey to wellness, we need to give ourselves a bit of a grace period to breathe and see the bigger picture.

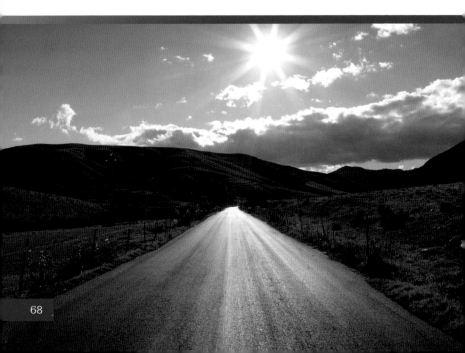

»Faith Life

Discouragement and setbacks are a part of life. Read Matthew 19:26. Do any of your goals feel impossible? Have you experienced setbacks? Go for a walk and try to grant yourself some grace as God grants grace to all of us.

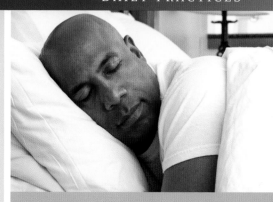

»Medical

Our medical model is often based on what we must *do*. Exercise, eat right, and take the right medications. But just as important is rest. Sleep gives the body enough energy to function healthfully. Today try to rest.

{
Wellness was about finding balance.
}

»Movement

Not all exercise must involve sweating! Today continue to work on your balance by spending ten minutes stretching. Try to touch your toes, get on the floor, stretch your back by pushing up on your arms, and reach each of your arms across your chest.

» Work

Do you work in an office where someone is always bringing in treats such as birthday cake, doughnuts, or bagels? Balance out some of these unhealthy snacks by bringing in a fruit plate to share. Maybe you'll inspire some healthier snacks next time!

» Emotional

When we're trying to establish new habits, it is easy to become overwhelmed, and in turn, to fall back on old, comfortable habits. Take a slow walk today, focusing on your breathing and letting go of the things that leave you feeling overwhelmed.

» Family and Friends

Family dinners are a wonderful place to begin wellness-oriented and balanced meals. Today plan a family dinner that contains mostly vegetables, a reasonable serving size of protein (like a lean meat), and a small serving of whole grains (rice, barley, or whole-wheat pasta).

» Nutrition

Depriving yourself entirely of the foods you love is more likely to push you to binge. Balance strict food intake and calorie counting with an occasional small treat. Treat yourself to a sensible treat today, such as a scoop of low-fat frozen yogurt or a cup of raspberries.

Evening Wrap-Up

As we continue on this journey toward wellness and weight management, we will encounter bumps in the road. When we encounter these obstacles, it can be all too easy to get discouraged, beating ourselves up (and others) for not necessarily sticking to the path. But we are assured daily that God offers us grace and abundant love. On this journey, we need to find ways to give grace to ourselves.

In you, LORD my God, I put my trust. . . . Show me your ways, LORD, teach me your paths. Guide me in your truth and teach me, for you are God my Savior, and my hope is in you all day long. Remember, LORD, your great mercy and love, for they are from of old. . .according to your love remember me, for you, LORD, are good.

PSALM 25: 1, 4–7

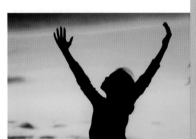

Gracious Lord, thank You for Your abundant grace and love. Help me today to give myself space to learn and grow on this journey. In Your holy name, Amen.

Morning Reflection

This week we are seeking balance in all aspects of our lives. So often, we can find ourselves in the mindset that weight management is about deprivation. We believe that we can only eat one kind of food or engage in one type of activity. But this week we are learning that when we live a balanced lifestyle, we actually incorporate many experiences from all our senses. After all, God has blessed us with the senses of sight, smell, sound, taste, and touch. It makes sense, then, that a wellness-oriented lifestyle includes all our senses.

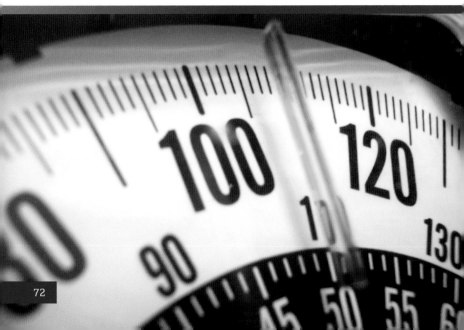

» Faith Life

Psalm 34:8 says, "Taste and see that the LORD is good; blessed is the one who takes refuge in him." Today say a prayer before every meal. Remember that God shows up in every aspect of our lives, including our food.

» Medical

An underlying medical condition can make weight management difficult. If you have tried to implement lifestyle changes and have seen negative outcomes, make sure that you talk to your doctor. Many such conditions can be managed or resolved.

» Movement

Today try to embrace all your senses as you go for a walk around your neighborhood. Observe all the colors, smells, and even tastes as you walk. But mostly, feel the air on your skin and feel the movement in your body.

» Work

We often focus on the negative effects of work, but working—being active and positively engaged—is an important component of wellness. Today try to focus on the positive engagement in your work—whether you work in an office or at home.

» Emotional

Emotions always have a significant effect on wellness, both for better and for worse. Sometimes emotions can get out of control, and we can lose perspective on the big picture. Today go for a walk and reflect on your "big picture." What is important to you? What is not?

» Family and Friends

Healthy relationships can bring balance to your life in many ways, but especially by offering fellowship and fun. Call a friend or a family member today and have some fun by dancing to some music or shopping at a farmer's market for some local fresh produce.

» Nutrition

Healthy food, especially when you use fresh ingredients and healthy spices, does not need to taste bad. Today make a meal using fresh vegetables, healthy fats, and lean proteins. Don't forget to season it with some fresh herbs!

Evening Wrap-Up

Then God said, "I give you every seed-bearing plant on the face of the whole earth and every tree that has fruit with seed in it. They will be yours for food. And to all the beasts of the earth and all the birds in the sky and all the creatures that move along the ground—everything that has the breath of life in it—I give every green plant for food." And it was so.

GENESIS 1:29–30

When we see, smell, and taste the world that God has created, we know that God has filled the world with beauty. God created us to be able to experience that beauty, and so we should participate in that beauty on our journey to wellness. When we live wellness-oriented lives, we live in the balance of all God's creation!

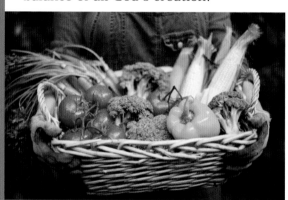

Loving God, You have filled my life with beautiful colors and delicious tastes and smells. Help me to live my life in the fullness of Your creation by taking the time to notice the wonder You have created around me. In Your holy name, Amen.

Morning Reflection

Most of us have pretty well-defined areas in which we are definitely comfortable and definitely uncomfortable. We have habits and patterns that are very comfortable and very difficult to break. Change is uncomfortable. But as we move forward on this journey, we can realize the discomfort that comes with change is also the discomfort that comes with growth, and God is with us as much in the uncomfortable changing zone as in the comfort zone.

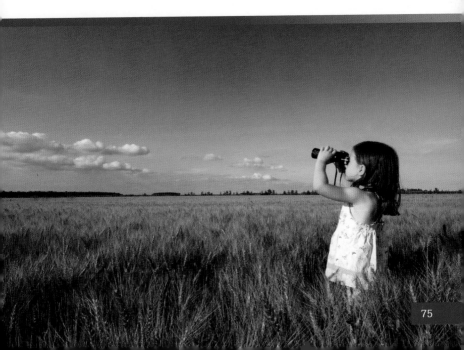

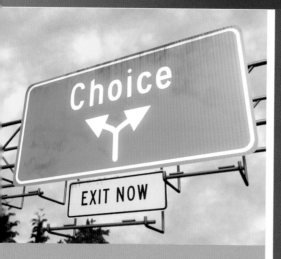

Have you ever felt called to leave your comfort zone? How did you handle it? Do you feel that God walked with you? Spend five minutes today meditating on how God has acted in your life outside of your comfort zone.

»Medical

Do you know the symptoms of stroke? They include weakness in an arm, hand, or leg; loss of feeling on one side of the body; blindness in one eye; difficulty talking; loss of balance. If you or someone you know experiences any of these symptoms, you should seek medical attention. Today take time to identify a local hospital or physician that you trust in the event an emergency happens in your family. Preparation is key.

»Movement

A healthy exercise regimen consists of building our aerobic strength, muscular strength, endurance, and flexibility. Today do three sets of ten wall push-ups to start building your upper-body strength.

Change is uncomfortable. But as we move forward on this journey. . .

»Work

Good posture helps you to breathe, increases strength in your back and ab-domen, and can help decrease back pain and headaches. Today at work, remind yourself to keep your head up and your shoulders back and relaxed.

»Emotional

At a time when you are not experiencing anxiety, make a plan for days when you feel overwhelmed. Select a Bible verse (or multiple Bible verses) to keep close at hand or identify friends or family that you can call for encouragement.

»Family and Friends

It can be less intimidating to leave your comfort zone if you have family and friends to do it with you. Today go for a walk with a friend or member of your family. Try to walk farther and at a more brisk pace than you usually do.

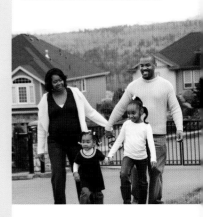

»Nutrition

Developing healthy eating habits can mean leaving behind food habits that have been comfortable for a long time. Today be particularly mindful of portion size as you eat. For example, a serving of meat should only be about the size of a deck of cards.

Evening Wrap-Up

Paul certainly knew about being forced out of his comfort zone.

In his letter to the Corinthians, Paul writes of moving out of his comfort zone in service of God. As we continue on this journey, we can take Paul's example and realize that change is not always going to be comfortable. But moving forward, we can know that God walks with us and continues to care for us when we leave our comfort zone.

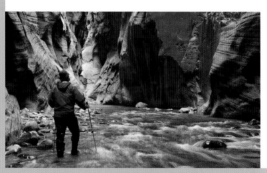

We put no stumbling block in anyone's path, so that our ministry will not be discredited. Rather, as servants of God we commend ourselves in every way: in great endurance; in troubles, hardships and distresses. . .known yet regarded as unknown; dying, and yet we live on; beaten, and yet not killed; sorrowful, yet always rejoicing; poor, yet making many rich; having nothing, and yet possessing everything.

2 CORINTHIANS 6:3–4, 9–10

Lord God, give me courage and encouragement to make the changes that I need to make in my life, even as I leave my comfort zone. In Your holy name, Amen.

Morning Reflection

At the beginning of the journey, we set both short-term and long-term goals so that we could measure our progress. As we approach the midpoint of our wellness journey, we need to take some time to revisit the purpose that we set up in the first week. Periodically revisiting our purpose can help us to balance our everyday frustrations with the bigger picture. Remember that the purpose is different from person to person, and may even change from day to day.

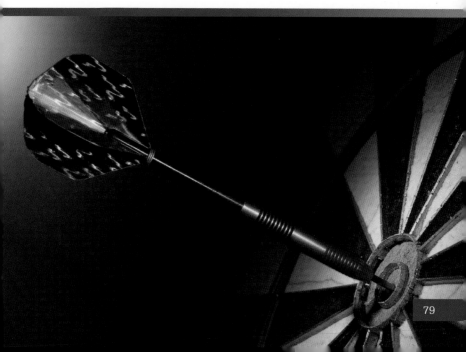

» Faith Life

Do you remember what your goals were for your faith life in week one? Today go back and read your goals, and then write for five minutes about your progress. Are your goals still the same? Have you made any unexpected progress?

» Medical

Do you know your family medical history? If your parents, grandparents, aunts, or uncles have or had an illness, it can be relevant to your own health. Along with your list of medications, include a family history of major medical problems.

» Movement

We all like to relax by watching television or reading a book. But that must be balanced by some kind of movement. Today while you watch television, try doing some bicep curls with hand weights or do several sets of squats.

» Work

Take a copy of that list of medications, vitamins, over-the-counter medications, and family history to keep at work. Also, if possible, have a place at work where you can keep the medication that you need during the day, instead of taking your medication with you to work every day.

» Emotional

Going through periods of change can be particularly taxing on our emotions. Connecting with our purpose can help us gain some stability. Today spend ten minutes writing in your journal about your purpose in this wellness journey.

» Family and Friends

Family and friends can be one of the strongest reminders of our purpose that we have. Today have a healthy meal with your family or some friends and enjoy the social anchor that you have in your support system.

» Nutrition

Instead of a cooked appetizer, try putting out some sliced-up fruits and vegetables. Instead of a cream or mayonnaise-based dipping sauce (like french onion or ranch dressing), try serving hummus or baba ghanoush.

Evening Wrap-Up

The journey toward wellness is a lifelong journey, and our purpose is what keeps us anchored. During our first week, we named our purpose. The journey toward weight management and wellness can be a frustrating one at times, and keeping an eye on our purpose can help us to balance the frustration with peace. Isaiah reminds us, too, that whatever our purpose, God holds us and offers us lasting peace.

Who has measured the waters in the hollow of his hand, or with the breadth of his hand marked off the heavens? Who has held the dust of the earth in a basket, or weighed the mountains on the scales and the hills in a balance?

Isaiah 40:12

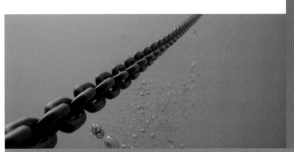

Loving God, help me to keep an eye on my purpose on this journey and to keep in mind that You are holding me in Your hand even now. In Your holy name, Amen.

Morning Reflection

This journey toward wellness and weight management is all about making changes. The problem is that change—even change that we want—can be challenging and stressful. In fact, as we work to make many changes at the same time, we can end up feeling thrown off-kilter. We can lose touch with our center and forget which way is "up." So today we will focus on how to stay balanced in the midst of all this change.

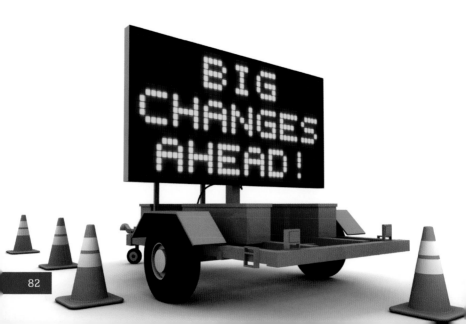

»Faith Life

Do you have a Bible verse or a special prayer that helps you to anchor your faith life? Today, spend ten minutes and reflect on that one verse or prayer that "anchors" you, even as you have been on this journey full of change. Consider writing the verse on a slip of paper or a card and taping it where you are sure to see it when you need it.

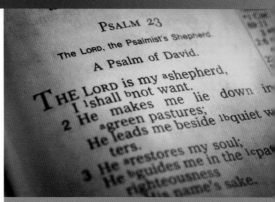

»Medical

If you are struggling to manage your weight, do you find yourself obsessing about food? Do you go on "binges" where you eat very large amounts of food? Do you exercise excessively? These are all symptoms of disordered eating and can lead to very serious health problems. If you experience any of these, talk to a doctor or a counselor immediately.

{ Focus on how to stay balanced in the midst of all this change. }

»Movement

When you go to the grocery store, once you have loaded up your cart, take an extra walk around the store. It won't take you much time, and it will add another hundred or so steps to your day (depending on the size of your grocery store!).

» Work

When work becomes topsy-turvy, it can be very easy to stress-eat without even recognizing what you are doing. Today if you start to feel overwhelmed at work, don't head for the vending machines, head for the door! Take a short break outside, breathe in some fresh air, and let your body relax before getting back to work.

» Emotional

How have you dealt with change in the past? Have you been able to embrace change? Or do you usually resist change? Go for a walk today, and take a different route than you usually do. Reflect on how you feel when you are trying something different.

» Family and Friends

Do your friends and family help anchor you? Let them know how important they are to you today. Write them a note, e-mail, or text message, or just call them on the phone.

» Nutrition

Salads are definitely healthy, but be careful of the dressing and cheese! Use lowfat cheese and substitute cream-based or mayonnaise-based dressings (like Ranch or Thousand Island) with a vinaigrette or even just some vinegar and oil with a little pepper and oregano.

Evening Wrap-Up

While change happens, and while we work to make positive change in our lives, we know that there is a constant. Even at those times when we feel things are the most topsy-turvy, we can rest in the knowledge that God is walking this journey with us, and God is constant and unchanging. The author of the letter to the Hebrews reminds us that all things change—even the heavens and the earth will wear out. But God remains steady and constant.

"In the beginning, Lord, you laid the foundations of the earth, and the heavens are the work of your hands. They will perish, but you remain; they will all wear out like a garment. You will roll them up like a robe; like a garment they will be changed. But you remain the same, and your years will never end."

HEBREWS 1:10–12

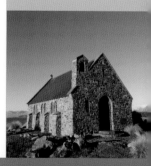

Loving God, I know that You are my constant. You are my rock. Today, remind me that You are my anchor even in the midst of change and chaos. In Your holy name, Amen.

Morning Reflection

At the end of this week, we are halfway through the six weeks. Congratulations! Sometimes at the halfway point, we might be able to see progress, and we may also look ahead and feel like there is still so much progress to be made. It is easy now to run out of steam—to lose momentum. But we are in the middle of the race, and it is now that we need to dig deep and tap into our extra stores of endurance to continue on the journey.

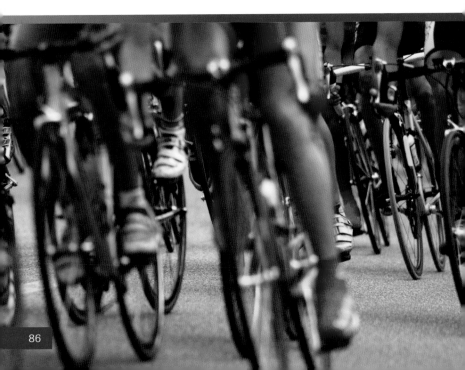

»Faith Life

Endurance requires, among other things, concentration. Today spend five minutes sitting quietly. Reflect on the journey to this point, and how God has been present with you.

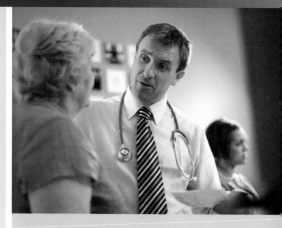

»Medical

Keep in mind that quick fixes in medicine are generally not good long-term solutions. The next time you have a doctor's appointment, talk to your care provider about your long-term health goals.

»Movement

To build endurance, you need to occasionally push your limits. Today do as many jumping jacks as you can, take a one-minute break, and then do it again. Try that three times throughout the day.

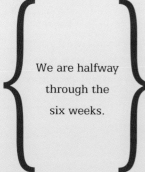

We are halfway through the six weeks.

»Work

Do you notice a time of day when you get hungry? Do you crave a specific food when you take your break? This may be habitual eating. Today when you feel hungry at work, drink some water, or snack on some carrot sticks instead of heading for the doughnuts or vending machines.

»Emotional

Marathon runners will tell you that endurance is at least as emotional as it is physical. Today spend five minutes breathing and repeat to yourself that you can. . . Can. . .CAN continue on this journey.

»Family and Friends

Who is your oldest friend? Sometimes the relationships we have had the longest are the easiest to neglect. Take time today to think of a long-term friend whom you have not spoken to in a while and drop him or her a line.

»Nutrition

Tonight for dessert, make fruit kebabs and serve them with some low-fat yogurt or cottage or ricotta cheese instead of making a sugar-rich and fatty dessert.

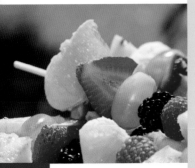

Evening Wrap-Up

As we stand at the halfway point of our journey, we can feel a whole host of emotions, ranging from celebration of the last few weeks to dread at what is yet to come. We may feel both proud and intimidated. This range of emotions is natural. Whatever our emotional state right now, we can take encouragement from Zechariah, who writes that the Lord will live among us. God walks this journey with us, celebrating with us and encouraging us when we feel discouraged.

"Shout and be glad, Daughter Zion. For I am coming, and I will live among you," declares the LORD. *"Many nations will be joined with the LORD in that day and will become my people. I will live among you and you will know that the LORD Almighty has sent me to you."*

ZECHARIAH 2:10–11

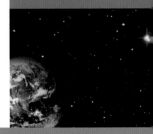

Loving God, I know that You have made me. As I strive to care for my body and spirit, I pray that You would guide me and encourage me on the journey. In Your holy name, Amen.

Church Health Center Wellness prides itself on being more than just a gym. It is a community center

that cares for the whole person, and no one better represents this spirit of wholeness than Tammy. After years of dealing with physical and emotional problems, Tammy says that she was look-ing for one person to tell her she was worth saving. But when she came to Church Health Center Wellness, she said she found more than one person. Instead, she found "a whole building full."

Both Tammy and her family had resigned themselves to life with severe obesity. She often rode a cart around the grocery store and had trouble getting out of bed. Her daughter took to making most of Tammy's clothes because it was difficult to find appropriate clothes that were affordable. When she first came to Wellness, Tammy was so obese it was difficult and often painful for her to exercise.

Because of her weight, she started on her road to health by taking classes in the therapeutic pool, where the warm waters supported her weight and eased the pain in her joints. Once she had built up her muscles and began losing weight, she moved on to the Sports Court where several wellness coordinators pushed her to reach her goals. Once she started working out regularly, she looked into our healthy kitchen and reinvented the way she thought about food. She even began attending our prayer services and volunteering in other ways at the Church Health Center.

Tammy worked her way through almost every program at the Wellness Center, taking classes, exercising, and volunteering her way back to health.

40 Days to Better Living

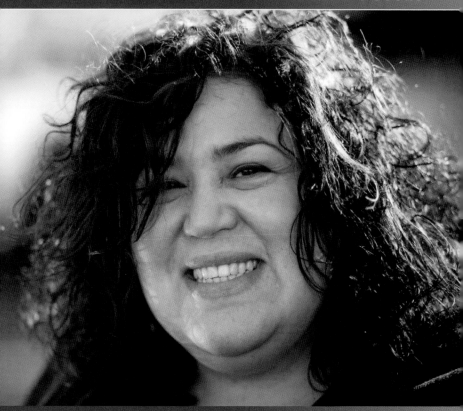

After years of dealing with physical and emotional problems, Tammy says that she was looking for one person to tell her she was worth saving. But when she came to Church Health Center Wellness. . .she found "a whole building full."

Morning Reflection

Have you ever watched a beautiful sunset and marveled at the wonders of God's creation? Many of us take the time to observe the wonders of God's creation in the world. But how many of us spend time standing in front of the mirror observing the wonders of God's creation in each of us? We might look at the bigger picture but miss the time to remember that we are each a part of God's wonderful creation. This week we will develop our understanding of God's creation, paying special attention to the place of our own bodies and spirits in creation.

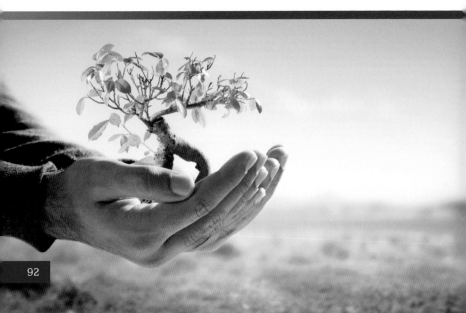

»Faith Life

All of creation belongs to God, though it can be easy to forget that. Today go for a prayerful walk and remember that the air that you breathe and the ground on which you walk belong to God.

»Medical

Good medicine is preventative medicine. This week we will focus on how to practice good preventative medicine at home. Today make a list of the ways that you take care of yourself on a weekly or monthly basis.

»Movement

A wonderful way to get some exercise and appreciate God's creation is to go for a hike. Find a park in your area that has some trails available to hike. Don't forget to bring water and a healthy snack.

{ . . .God's creation, paying special attention to the place of our own bodies and spirits in creation. }

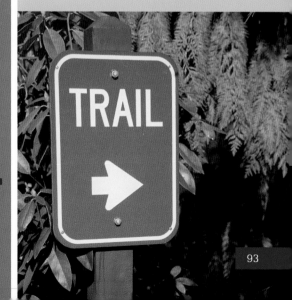

93

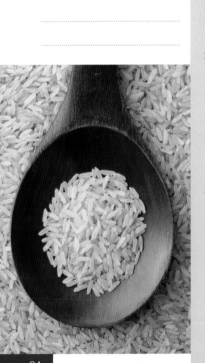

»Work

Being trapped inside all day can lead to some considerable burnout if you don't take time outside at some point. Today before work or after work, find five minutes to spend outside.

»Emotional

Practice slow, deep breathing today. Relax your shoulders, lift your chin, close your eyes, and take a deep breath using your abdominal muscles. Breathe in through your nose, hold your breath in for three seconds, then slowly let your breath out through your mouth.

»Family and Friends

Picnics are a wonderful way to connect with your family and friends. Today go on a picnic with your friends and family. Instead of hot dogs and hamburgers, pack fresh fruit, lean meats, and low-fat cheeses.

»Nutrition

This week, we are going to focus on how to make your calories count. The first step is to eat whole grains. Buy whole-grain, low-fat breads, snack crackers, and pasta. Use brown rice instead of white rice.

Evening Wrap-Up

We know, from the very first chapter of Genesis, the amount of care and love that God has put into creation is great. But even as we notice the care and power that has gone into all of creation, it is worth noticing that the love and care that goes into a majestic sunset is the same love and care that goes into each of us.

How many are your works, LORD! In wisdom you made them all; the earth is full of your creatures. There is the sea, vast and spacious, teeming with creatures beyond number—living things both large and small. There the ships go to and fro, and Leviathan, which you formed to frolic there . . . . May the glory of the LORD endure forever. . .he who looks at the earth, and it trembles, who touches the mountains, and they smoke.

PSALM 104:24–26, 31–32

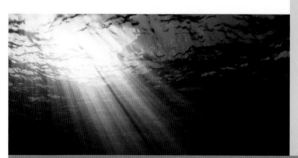

God of creation, thank You for opening my eyes to the beauty of creation. Help me to remember that I, too, am a part of Your creation. In Your holy name, Amen.

95

Morning Reflection

The sun is one aspect of God's creation that we often take for granted. After all, the sun is there each morning. It is often hot and occasionally a nuisance. Most of us spend most (if not all) of our time indoors, and the sun has become somewhat scary in our consciousness. But the truth is, healthy sun exposure can help to lift our mood and can give us more energy. Healthy interaction with the sun can really help us on this weight-management journey.

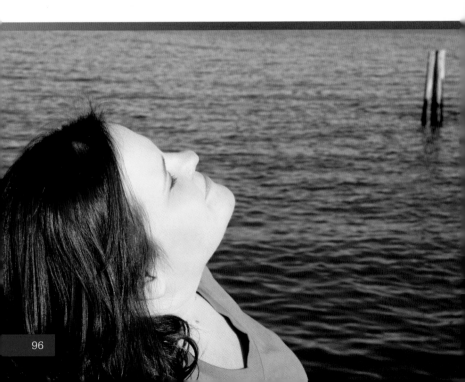

»Faith Life

When you walk out into the sun, do you think of God? Today when you have the sun in your eyes or you walk outside into the sunshine, say a brief prayer. "Thank You, God, for the sunshine."

{ Healthy interaction with the sun can really help us. }

»Medical

Though exposure to the sun is important, overexposure to the sun can cause serious health problems. Today check your body for moles and spots, using the ABCD rule. If the mole is asymmetric, has irregular borders, has a variation in color, or has a diameter larger than a pencil eraser, you should get it checked by your health care provider.

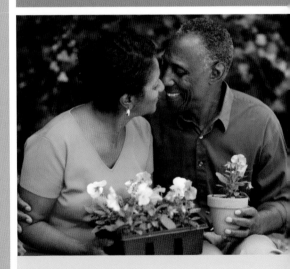

»Movement

Spend some time outside today, walking or even going for a light jog. Remember to put on sunblock before you spend any significant amount of time outside.

97

» Work

Enjoying the sun can be particularly difficult at our jobs, but our work is not just at our job. Today do some work outside. Wash your car, mow your lawn, or work in your garden.

» Emotional

The sun can provide a much-needed emotional lift, as well as vitamin D. Find ten minutes today to sit outside in the sun and practice deep breathing. Feel the sun's warmth, and try to let your body relax as you sit.

» Family and Friends

How often do you gather your family and friends for any kind of outdoor activity? Today plan an outdoor social activity with your family and friends, even if it is only eating dinner outside.

» Nutrition

Do you eat cereal in the morning? Instead of a sweetened cereal, choose an unsweetened, whole-grain cereal and sweeten it with cut fruit, such as bananas or berries. If you must have your cereal sweetened further, use an artificial sweetener.

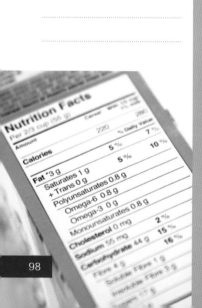

Evening Wrap-Up

We are told that the first moment of God's creation was light. God

created the sun, giving us a wonderful gift that is beautiful, and that offers joy and health (when used correctly). There are many of us who get so busy with our lives that we forget to step out into the sun. We don't give our bodies the gift of safely enjoying the light and warmth that are products of this first gift of God's creation. The truly amazing thing is, if we do enjoy God's creation responsibly, we will also be healthier.

And God said, "Let there be light," and there was light. God saw that the light was good, and he separated the light from the darkness. God called the light "day," and the darkness he called "night." And there was evening, and there was morning— the first day.

GENESIS 1:3–5

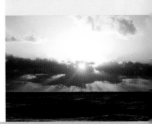

Living Light, thank You for Your gift of the sun. Help me to enjoy and appreciate the light that You have offered all of us. In Your holy name, Amen.

Morning Reflection

The very first thing many of us do when we wake in the morning is to yawn and stretch. We take in a breath. Our bodies breathe without our even thinking about it. Generally, we only notice the air if it smells bad or if there is not enough of it. But the air is such a beautiful and important part of God's creation. So today we are going to focus on ways to be healthier with the air.

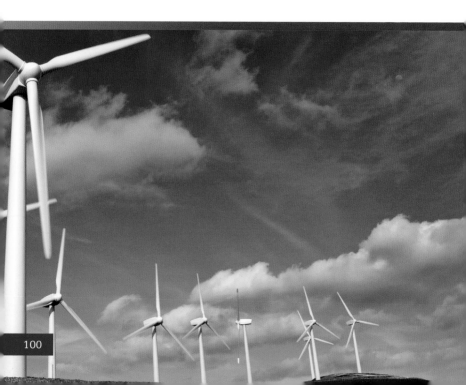

» Faith Life

There are dozens of verses in the Bible about how God uses the wind. Today read John 3:8, and when you encounter the wind today, take it as a reminder of God's Spirit moving in the world.

» Medical

Cigarette smoking greatly inhibits your ability to breathe. If you do smoke, talk to your primary care provider about ways to help you quit. Smoking simply does not have a place in wellness.

» Movement

When you walk, do you walk fast enough to feel the wind on your face or hair? Today try scattering some "walking sprints" throughout your walk—walk at a normal pace for two minutes, then at a much faster pace for thirty seconds, and repeat. This will help you get your heart rate up, and you'll get more out of your walk.

» Work

If you feel anxiety at work, try to do some deep breathing. Breathe in through your nose and out through your mouth. You do not need to do this for extended periods of time at work. Simply give yourself a few breaths to relax.

» Emotional

Air is a very important part of stress relief. Today spend five minutes sitting with your back straight, breathing. Breathe in through your nose and out through your mouth. If you start to feel lightheaded, try to relax your chest and stomach muscles.

» Family and Friends

Today go on a walk with a friend or family member, but try to remain silent during the walk. Try to enjoy the silence and company of your friend and concentrate on your breathing, enjoying the fresh air. After the walk, talk with your friend about how he or she enjoyed the "silent walk."

» Nutrition

Avoid vegetables that are fried or prepared in heavy cream sauces or butter. Instead, bake your vegetables (such as squash and potatoes) or steam them (broccoli, asparagus, green beans).

Evening Wrap-Up

And God said, "Let there be a vault between the waters to separate water from water." So God made the vault and separated the water under the vault from the water above it. And it was so. God called the vault "sky." And there was evening, and there was morning—the second day.

GENESIS 1:6–8

On this weight-management

journey, we are working to gain more appreciation for our bodies. That means, among other things, recognizing that we are as much a part of God's great creation as the fresh air that we inhale. So today as we take a breath and acknowledge that which gives us life, let us also notice that our bodies are doing the breathing. We are intimately tied up with every aspect of God's creation.

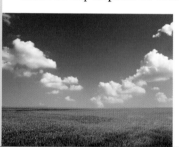

Loving God, thank You for giving me breath. Help me today to truly notice the beauty of the very air that I breathe. In Your holy name, Amen.

Morning Reflection

Water is crucial for life. It covers about 70 percent of the earth's surface, and our own bodies are made up of about 57 percent water on average. But most health experts make it fairly clear that, generally speaking, we are not drinking enough water, which can lead to a myriad of health problems. At the most basic level, the path to wellness and weight management is paved with water, so today we will focus on the significant role that water plays in our wellness and weight-management journey.

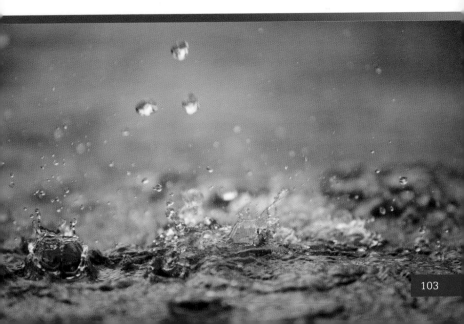

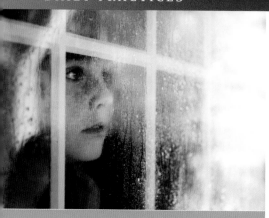

»Faith Life

How often have we complained when it starts raining? Today write a prayer thanking God for the rain and for all of the ways that you are thankful for water in your life.

»Medical

Try drinking cold water rather than luke-warm water. When our bodies warm up cold water to our body temperature, we actually burn additional calories.

»Movement

Swimming is excellent exercise. It is gentle on your joints and works just about every muscle group in your body. Today if you have access to a pool, go for a swim— even spending ten minutes in the water will give you some great exercise.

{ The path to wellness is paved with water. }

»Work

Bring a refillable water bottle to work. When you are feeling thirsty, or craving a soda, fill up your water bottle and sip from the bottle throughout the day. Staying hydrated will help you keep your energy level up and will keep you from drinking sugary sodas.

»Emotional

Most of us shower in the morning. Today take a five-minute shower at the end of the day to warm your muscles and relax.

»Family and Friends

Serving water with meals is a great way to meet your daily fluid goals (about eight 8-ounce glasses). Today serve water instead of soda or other sweetened beverages.

»Nutrition

If you want a beverage other than water, drink some unsweetened herbal tea or fruit juice, but stick with 100 percent fruit juice. Also, try to get more of your fruit servings every day from whole fruit rather than juice.

And God said, "Let the water under the sky be gathered to one place, and let dry ground appear." And it was so. God called the dry ground "land," and the gathered waters he called "seas." And God saw that it was good.

GENESIS 1:9–10

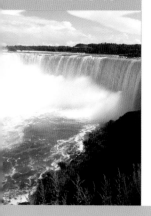

Evening Wrap-Up

God created the earth and made water cover the majority of the

surface of the planet. Furthermore, our very bodies are composed mostly of water. Water also plays an important role throughout scripture. In 1 Kings 17, we hear about a devastating drought, and then we hear about the destructive power of water in the story of Noah's ark. Water reveals both God's care for us and the power of God's hand. So on this journey to wellness and weight management, we can remember that God's power—the power of water—is within each of us.

God of mercy, thank You for the gift of water. Help me today to remember that water is a crucial part of my body and of Your creation. In Your holy name, Amen.

Morning Reflection

When we think of God's creation, the first image that comes to mind is most often associated with the earth: lush, beautiful forests; alien-looking deserts; the Grand Canyon. This is the part of creation that provides us with the food to eat. The land is designed by God to give us a rich variety of foods, and yet many of us have very little connection to where much of our food comes from. Today we will turn our focus to this aspect of God's creation.

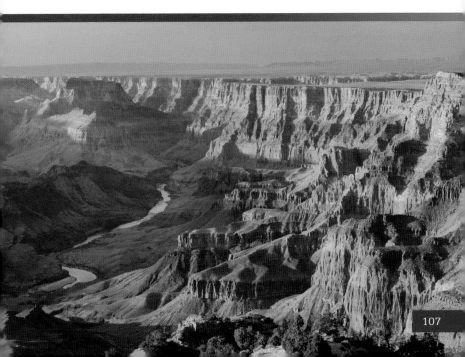

» Faith Life

When you sit down to eat a meal, do you see God's creation? When you sit down to meals today, try to imagine where each piece of your meal came from, and give thanks for each item.

» Medical

Losing weight rapidly can affect your muscle and bone mass. If you have recently lost a good deal of weight, talk to your doctor about ways that you can care for your bones and muscles even while you are losing weight.

» Movement

Gardening can provide great exercise. If you do not have the space to have a full garden, try planting some tomatoes or herbs in pots.

» Work

Do your coworkers know about your journey to wellness? Today tell at least one of your coworkers about your journey. Often workplaces can come together to strive toward wellness as a community.

» Emotional

Being a member of a community is a very important part of emotional wellness as well as physical wellness. Today spend at least ten minutes talking with a member of your support system.

» Family and Friends

A farmer's market can be a great way to find affordable local produce, and it can be a great place to spend some time with friends and family. Today take a few minutes and see if your town has a farmer's market.

» Nutrition

The more fresh your food, the healthier it is. If you cannot find a vegetable in the fresh produce section, try the frozen food section. "Flash frozen" fruits and vegetables are just as nutritious as fresh vegetables and can be used in the same recipes.

Evening Wrap-Up

We can look out our window and see the remarkable gift of God's

creation in the grass, the trees, and the flowers. But what about when we open our refrigerators? How about when we sit down to dinner? Do we see God's creation? If we did see God's creation in our meals, would we eat differently? God cares for us by offering us all different aspects of creation: water, air, and land.

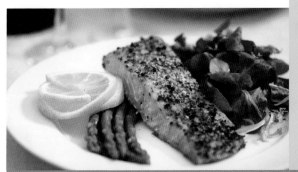

Then God said, "Let the land produce vegetation: seed-bearing plants and trees on the land that bear fruit with seed in it, according to their various kinds." And it was so. The land produced vegetation: plants bearing seed according to their kinds and trees bearing fruit with seed in it according to their kinds. And God saw that it was good. And there was evening, and there was morning— the third day.

GENESIS 1:11–13

Loving God, thank You for the gift that You have given me in Your creation. Help me to see Your hand at work each day. In Your holy name, Amen.

Morning Reflection

We often forget that our bodies are as much a part of creation as the breeze blowing through the trees. As we started this weight-management journey, many of us did not have a loving relationship with our bodies. But as the psalmist reminds us, each of us was stitched together in our mother's womb (Psalm 139:13). Because of the care that God has put into creating us, our bodies deserve the same reverence that we show to the rest of God's creation.

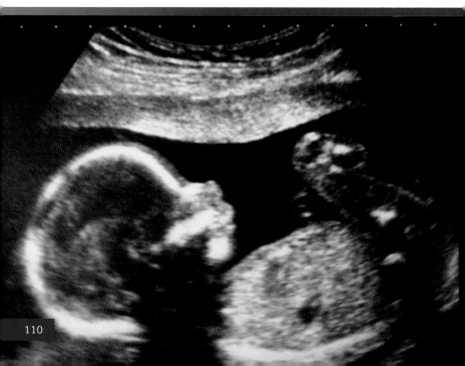

»Faith Life

Today at the time when you pray, pray a movement prayer. Stretch out your arms. Touch your toes. Stretch your neck. Feel the brilliance in God's creation and the way that your body is put together.

{ We are created to be social beings, not isolated from one another.

»Medical

If you do not give yourself a monthly breast exam or testicular exam, today is the day to start. Finding breast cancer and testicular cancer early greatly increases the chances of recovery.

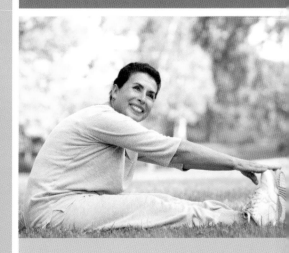

»Movement

Today go for a brisk walk, and when you are finished, spend at least five minutes stretching. Try to feel and stretch as many muscles in your body as possible.

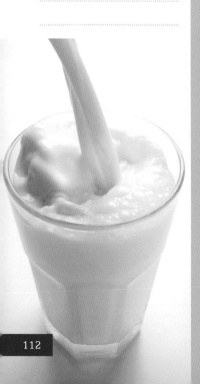

» Work

Work often requires repetitive motion.
When you take a break, spend five minutes
doing something completely different than
what you usually do. For example, if you sit
at a computer typing most of the day, stand
up and do jumping jacks.

» Emotional

**Our emotions are more tied up with our
bodies than we usually realize.** Today
spend five minutes smiling, even if you do not
feel like smiling. Chances are you will feel a
little better at the end of those five minutes.

» Family and Friends

**Many of our self-esteem issues stem from
directing hatred toward our own bodies.**
Today ask a friend or family member to tell
you what he or she likes about your body.

» Nutrition

Include three calcium-rich products today.
Low-fat dairy can be part of a healthy diet.

Evening Wrap-Up

During the first week, we noted the importance of our own "fleshy" bodies, noting especially how "flesh" gets a bad rap. But in this passage from the Gospel of John, we see that, not only did God come "in the flesh," as Jesus, but He did it twice! John makes a special point of making sure we know that Jesus ate breakfast when He showed up after the resurrection, meaning His body was a real, fleshy body. God values the body enough to keep it, even after death!

Jesus said to them, "Come and have breakfast." None of the disciples dared ask him, "Who are you?" They knew it was the Lord. Jesus came, took the bread and gave it to them, and did the same with the fish. This was now the third time Jesus appeared to his disciples after he was raised from the dead.

JOHN 21:12–14

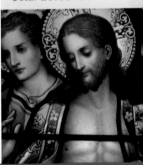

Loving God, give me the vision to see my body as a gift from You and the strength to care for my body, just as You care for all of creation. In Your holy name, Amen.

Morning Reflection

On this journey, we have already established that God has created each of us whole—body and spirit.

But today, as we reach the final day of the fourth week, we can come to acknowledge that our spirits are a very important part of God's creation that work in concert with the rest of creation. Though we often think of "health" as being primarily about the body, our spirits are central to wellness. Today we will focus on how our spirits contribute to our overall wellness.

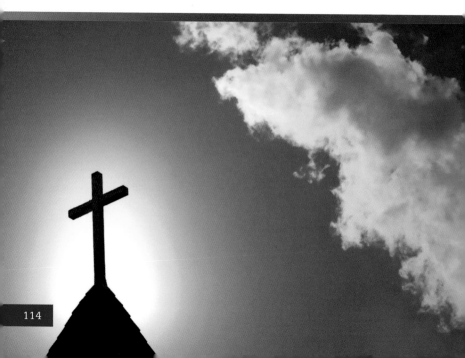

»Faith Life

How would you describe a healthy spirit? Take ten minutes today to pray and then write a few sentences about what a healthy spirit means to you.

{ Today we will focus on how our spirits contribute to our overall wellness. }

»Medical

Today make a list of things you need to discuss with your health care provider next time you visit his or her office.

»Movement

Helping a neighbor do yard work or even load a moving truck is a wonderful act of kindness and generosity, and it can get your heart rate up and burn calories, to boot! Today try to help a friend, family member, or neighbor with a project.

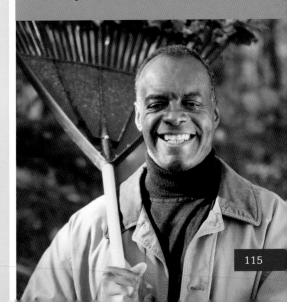

115

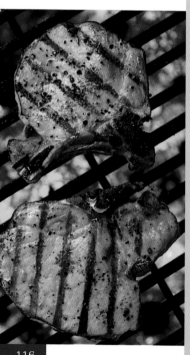

»Work

If you find yourself standing in one place for a period of time (making copies, talking on the phone, waiting for lunch to heat up), spend that time raising yourself onto your toes and then lowering yourself back down, increasing the strength in your calves.

»Emotional

We often expect perfection of ourselves. The trouble with such expectations is that we are simply not perfect, and we can become demoralized. Today write for ten minutes about a time that you have expected perfection from yourself.

»Family and Friends

Today recruit some family members and friends to help you with a project that you have been putting off—rearranging furniture, painting a room, mowing the lawn. Getting things accomplished is a great way to bond and lift spirits generally.

»Nutrition

When you cook meat, trim the visible fat before you cook it. Do not fry the meat—bake it or grill it. When it is cooked, drain the remaining fat.

Evening Wrap-Up

At this point in our journey, often we can start to notice a difference in our day-to-day lives. Perhaps we are not reaching as quickly for the bag of potato chips, or we are finding ways to add a few extra steps to each day. These changes may seem small, but when added together, they're significant steps on the weight-management journey. In his letter to the Galatians, Paul reminds us of the fruits of the Spirit. On our journey, the fruits of the Spirit that we are seeing are those extra steps.

But the fruit of the Spirit is love, joy, peace, forbearance, kindness, goodness, faithfulness, gentleness and self-control. Against such things there is no law. Those who belong to Christ Jesus have crucified the flesh with its passions and desires. Since we live by the Spirit, let us keep in step with the Spirit.

GALATIANS 5:22–25

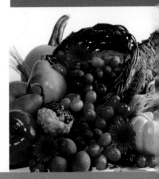

Dear Lord God, help me to see Your Spirit at work in me as I continue on this journey to wellness. In Your holy name, Amen.

James was a graduate student when he came to the Church Health Center about four years ago.

Because he was on a fixed income, he could not afford a gym membership. He felt discouraged and unhealthy, and he gained some weight. When he found that he could join Church Health Center Wellness for a reasonable fee, he joined on the spot.

He got connected with a wellness trainer and started not just exercising on a regular basis but also making important changes to his diet and lifestyle. He took classes that helped him find ways to make healthy lifestyle choices on a limited budget. Some of his favorite activities were the free cooking classes offered on Thursday nights and the guided relaxation classes on Monday mornings. Now, four years after he first joined, he has lost fifteen pounds and is maintaining his weight with his healthy lifestyle.

James now looks back on his journey and reflects on what he has learned. He says that while he had started his journey just looking for a place to work out, "I've learned that wellness is not just about exercise or belonging to a gym. It's about a whole lifestyle."

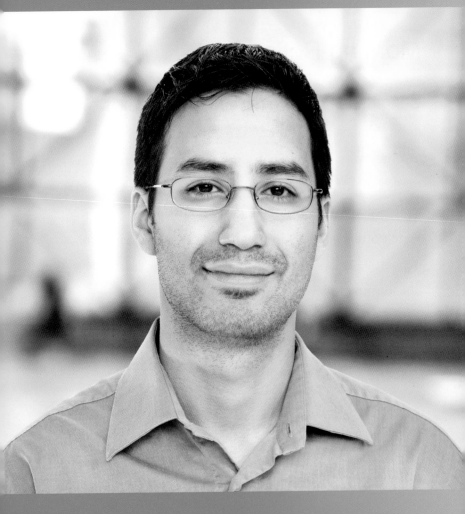

"I've learned that wellness is not just about exercise or belonging to a gym. It's about a whole lifestyle."

Weight Management

Morning Reflection

Congratulations! We have reached week five. At this point, we are beginning to see changes in ourselves and in our lifestyles. But as we progress on this journey to weight management, we are also seeing that the journey is not always consistent. Instead, it is an infinitely varied road, which often takes us in directions that we may not have expected. This week we will explore the many ways that our journey to weight management is full of variety.

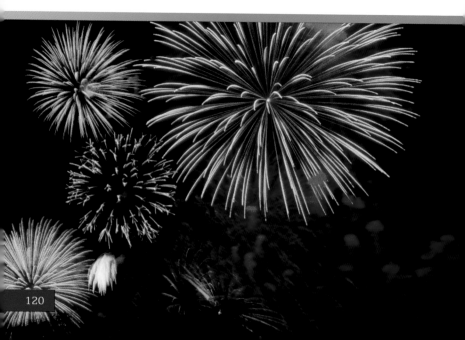

»Faith Life

Our faith journey, like our wellness journey, is a long and varied one. Spend ten minutes today writing about a time in your faith journey when you thought you were beginning one particular stage of a journey but ended up somewhere else entirely.

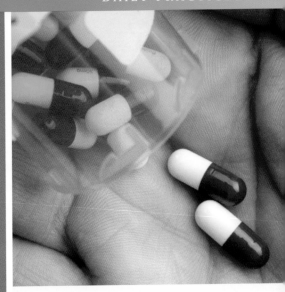

{ The journey is infinitely varied. }

»Medical

Are you taking medications? Have you been feeling better? Do not stop taking any medications until you have discussed it with your primary care provider. Stopping medication suddenly can lead to relapse, drug resistance, or unexpected side effects.

»Movement

Go for a walk in your neighborhood today. Take a coin and each time you arrive at a corner, flip the coin to decide whether to turn left or right.

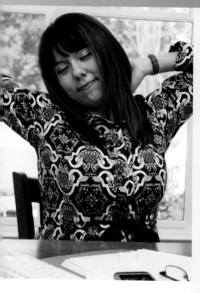

» Work

Each hour at work, take a minute or two just to stretch your arms and back. This will help keep you limber, and can help keep you focused throughout the day.

» Emotional

The unpredictability of our weight-management journey can sometimes feel overwhelming. Today make a list of what your expectations are at this point. Compare them with your expectations at the beginning of the journey.

» Family and Friends

Family and friends can be our constants when other things in life are unpredictable. Today make a healthy meal for your family or some friends. Enjoy the food, but focus on the company and conversation.

» Nutrition

Have you continued writing in your food journal throughout the journey? If not, start up again today. Keeping a journal of what you eat can really help to make you more aware of what you are eating every day.

Evening Wrap-Up

Last week we looked at God's creation and reflected on the wonders present in creation. Today we have taken a second look to notice the variety of color that is a part of that creation. King David illustrates just how many different colors are available and how beautiful the world is. This means that we can be reminded of God's presence each time we encounter something as simple as a differently colored stone. What a blessing!

"With all my resources I have provided for the temple of my God—gold for the gold work, silver for the silver, bronze for the bronze, iron for the iron and wood for the wood, as well as onyx for the settings, turquoise, stones of various colors, and all kinds of fine stone and marble—all of these in large quantities."

1 Chronicles 29:2

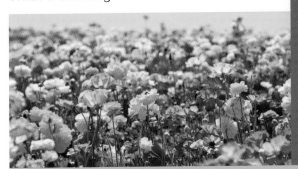

God of beauty, thank You for the journey that You have laid out for me. Help me today to embrace the journey, whatever the direction it takes me. In Your holy name, Amen.

Morning Reflection

A significant part of our weight-management journey has been reinterpreting our relationship with food. This has meant cutting back on certain kinds of food and finding ways to incorporate new foods into our diets. But how often do we stop and consider the wonder of the variety of tastes available to us each day? Today we will turn our focus to the way that God's care for us shines through the food that we eat.

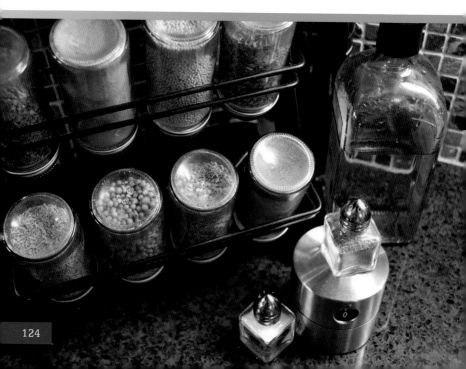

»Faith Life

Today each time you eat, give thanks for the food that God has given you. Try to pause even when you have a small snack to say a prayer.

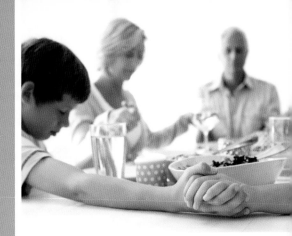

»Medical

At this point in your journey, you may be considering a more rigorous exercise routine. Remember to check in with your doctor and get a physical before beginning a rigorous exercise regimen.

»Movement

Today spend fifteen minutes doing abdominal-strength exercises. Standard sit-ups or crunches are a very good way to strengthen your body. Make sure that you don't strain your neck or back as you do those crunches!

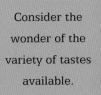

Consider the wonder of the variety of tastes available.

125

» Work

Instead of going out to eat or getting lunch out of a vending machine, bring in a lunch made from your leftovers from last night's dinner. It is almost guaranteed to be healthier, and it is much less expensive!

» Emotional

Give yourself a rest today. Spend a half hour doing something you really enjoy. Read a book, listen to music, watch a television show, or take a bath. Just take care of yourself for thirty minutes without worrying about the things that you "have to do."

» Family and Friends

Do you have friends or family who are somehow involved in this journey with you? If you don't, make a list today of potential friends or family members who might be a partner as you continue on the journey.

» Nutrition

Some fats are necessary for balanced nutrition. Healthy fats can be found in avocados, seeds and nuts, olive oil, and fish. Today prepare a meal using mostly healthy fats. (Avoid fried food or butter.)

Evening Wrap-Up

Each time we sit down to a meal,

we can truly taste and see that the Lord is good. When we bite into a tart apple or feel the heat of a jalapeño pepper on our tongue, we can taste the wonder and variety of God's creation. As we move forward, we can take full advantage of the variety of God's bounty. The more variety we take into our diet, the more healthy our lifestyle will be.

I will extol the LORD at all times; his praise will always be on my lips. I will glory in the LORD; let the afflicted hear and rejoice. Glorify the LORD with me; let us exalt his name together. . . . Taste and see that the LORD is good; blessed is the one who takes refuge in him.

PSALM 34:1–3, 8

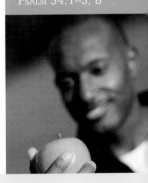

Lord God, thank You for the gift of new tastes. Help me to take refuge in You when I feel overwhelmed by the newness. In Your holy name, Amen.

Morning Reflection

At this point in our journey, we have experienced a variety of "seasons." We have experienced the beginning and the middle of this six-week journey, and we are approaching the end. We have gone through seasons of feeling encouraged and discouraged, seasons of feeling good, and seasons of feeling not so good. But it is important as we travel through these seasons, that we not give up on the journey altogether. Instead we must recognize that seasons require patience and perseverance. Today we will concentrate on the seasons that make up the journey.

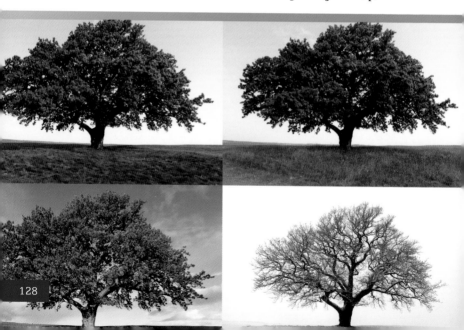

» Faith Life

What is your favorite season of the year? Spend five minutes writing about your favorite season. Then spend five minutes writing about your least favorite season. Can you find God both in your favorite and least favorite seasons?

» Medical

On this journey you have experienced a number of different and possibly new foods. Have you experienced any unusual reactions (stomach cramps, nausea, etc.) in response to those foods? That may indicate something as simple as an allergy. Check with your doctor at your next visit.

» Movement

Remember that you can walk outside whatever the season. Go for a walk outside today. If it's cold, wear a coat. If it's hot, wear shorts and a T-shirt. Try to enjoy the seasons that you experience.

» Work

Most workplaces have periods that are busy and periods that are slower. Whatever your work environment is like at this moment, find five minutes to breathe and stretch a little.

» Emotional

Are your expectations that your lifestyle changes will be all-or-nothing? Today take five minutes to write in your journal, reminding yourself that setbacks and individual "failures" are just seasons. If we persevere, they pass.

» Family and Friends

Ask one of the family members or friends on the list you made yesterday to be your "wellness buddy." Walking this journey without a partner can make a difficult journey even more difficult.

» Nutrition

Variety is the key to a balanced diet. Today prepare a meal that includes as many colors as you can fit into the meal. To easily add some variety, offer some raw, cut vegetables (such as carrot sticks or sliced red bell peppers) in addition to a cooked vegetable.

Evening Wrap-Up

There is a time for everything, and a season for every activity under the heavens: a time to be born and a time to die, a time to plant and a time to uproot, a time to kill and a time to heal, a time to tear down and a time to build, a time to weep and a time to laugh, a time to mourn and a time to dance, a time to scatter stones and a time to gather them, a time to embrace and a time to refrain from embracing.

ECCLESIASTES 3:1–5

Our weight-management journey

has already included and will continue to contain changes of seasons. But this is simply the result of the pattern of God's creation. God has built the changes of seasons into creation itself. But that does not necessarily make the changes that we encounter easy, even when those changes are welcomed.

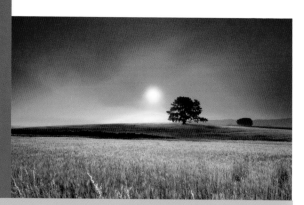

God in the midst of change, help me to embrace changes in my life as I move forward on this journey. In Your holy name, Amen.

Morning Reflection

Our wellness journey consists of not just differing seasons, but also many different sounds. Because the weight-management journey is about changing our entire lifestyle, it is only natural that some of the sounds we hear on a regular basis will change over time. We may even find ourselves speaking differently about wellness and our bodies. After all, James thought he just wanted to work out but found himself enjoying an entire lifestyle change.

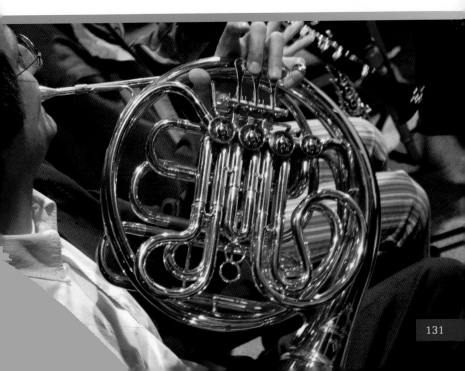

»Medical

On this journey to weight management, it is a good idea to keep tabs on your blood pressure. High blood pressure generally comes with no symptoms. So if you go to a drugstore today, check your blood pressure—just so that you can be aware of the number.

»Movement

Sound can be such an important part of movement, but we often ignore it. Today go for a walk and listen to the rhythm of your feet on the ground and the sound of your breath. You may even be able to hear your heartbeat as it rises.

»Faith Life

What is your favorite sound in the world? Today write for five minutes about that sound. What does the sound make you think of? Where does God fit into that sound?

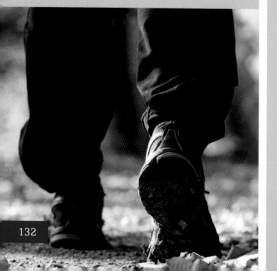

{
It is only natural that some of the sounds that we hear on a regular basis will change.
}

»Work

If you are able today, put on some soft music while you work, using either small speakers or headphones. Listening to music can help to pass time and can also lift your mood or relax you.

»Emotional

If you feel frustrated, try making some noise. Scream into a pillow or bang some pots and pans together. Making the noise will help you to relieve some aggression and frustration so you can gradually relax.

»Family and Friends

When you gather family and friends for a holiday or special occasion, think about playing games instead of focusing entirely on food. That way, the gathering is more about being in each others' company than eating.

»Nutrition

Instead of buying canned soup, make a large pot of soup on the stove top or using a slow cooker. Eat some tonight and put at least one night's worth in the freezer to eat on a busy day. Remember to season the soup with spices and herbs rather than with salt.

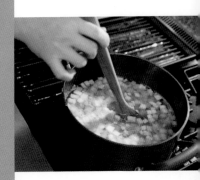

Evening Wrap-Up

Sound can be reminders of God's grace and presence in our lives. Noises can also be ways that we can praise and worship God. The psalmist writes, "Make a joyful noise." Can there be a more joyful noise than a healthy person moving and enjoying the movement? What would happen if we considered the sound of our feet on the pavement on the same level as praise and worship songs? We would probably walk a little more. As we move forward, let us remember that God loves us and wants us to be healthy.

Shout for joy to God, all the earth! Sing the glory of his name; make his praise glorious. Say to God, "How awesome are your deeds! . . . All the earth bows down to you. . .they sing the praises of your name."

PSALM 66:1–4

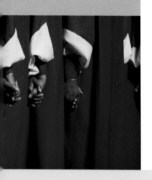

Loving God, thank You for the gift of sound. Help me to listen more carefully on this journey to weight management. In Your holy name, Amen.

Morning Reflection

The entire world is full of beautiful sights. On any given day there are many beautiful things to see. But on our journey to weight management, our eyesight, in a manner of speaking, might change. For example, food labels and methods of preparation that were once appealing may not look too appealing anymore. Driving our car to the corner market may look like a lost opportunity to take a nice walk. Wellness and the lifestyle that goes with it change our perspective in many ways.

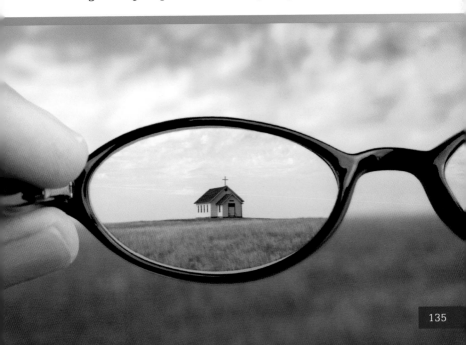

» Faith Life

Do you have potluck dinners at your church? The next time you have a potluck dinner, try bringing a healthy dish instead of a more typical dish. (For example, bring fresh fruit instead of a pie.)

» Medical

As you are making changes to your lifestyle, your body may respond in ways that you did not expect. But if you are consistently making changes and you feel worse, talk to your doctor.

» Movement

Go for a walk today. Walk for as long as you can manage and take in the sights of the world around you. Try to notice the difference in your walking now from when you started.

» Work

Protect yourself from picking up viruses at work by disinfecting your work space. If you work at a desk, remember to wipe down your phone and carefully clean your computer keyboard. If it is flu season, be sure to get a flu shot. Our places of work, as well as the gym, bus, or even our families, can be a hotbed for the flu virus. Avoid getting sick when you can so you can enjoy your progress on the journey.

» Emotional

Today, for comparison's sake, keep a log of your emotions throughout the day. Write when you feel happy, tired, frustrated, bored, and what you do (if anything) to deal with the emotion.

» Family and Friends

It can sometimes be difficult to reach out to family and friends when you need support. But today let one of your friends or family members know what kind of support you need on your wellness journey, even if they are not on the journey with you.

» Nutrition

If you are craving something sweet, eat a piece of fruit. If you really want a piece of candy or a sugary desert, try eating a small piece of dark chocolate. Dark chocolate has less fat and less sugar than milk chocolate.

Evening Wrap-Up

Before we make an effort to live wellness-oriented lives, it can be like living in blindness. But as we make progress toward wellness, our eyes are opened and we can see both who we are and how God relates to us in this journey. After all, God opens the eyes of the blind. God is forever faithful, and as we continue on this journey, we can lean on God, giving ourselves over to God's grace.

*How abundant are the good things that you have stored up for those who fear you, that you bestow in the sight of all, on those who take refuge in you. . . . Love the L*ORD*, all his faithful people! The L*ORD* preserves those who are true to him, but the proud he pays back in full. Be strong and take heart, all you who hope in the L*ORD*.*

PSALM 31:19, 23–24

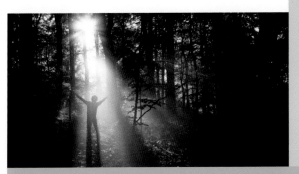

Loving God, grant me a new perspective as I continue on this journey to weight management. Help me to see Your hand at work in my life. In Your holy name, Amen.

Morning Reflection

The fruits of our journey are beginning to show up in our daily living. We are approaching the end of our six-week journey, and so we are seeing some small results. Perhaps we have reached some small goals, or we are getting close. But the true results will not really show themselves until we live our lives differently. That is the point of the journey: a changed life. The fruit of wellness-oriented weight management is, quite simply, life.

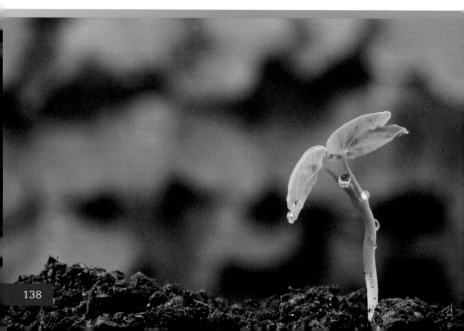

»Faith Life

Today spend five minutes meditating. Breathe deeply, quiet your "inner voices," and turn your focus to the wellness journey. Where have you felt God on the journey?

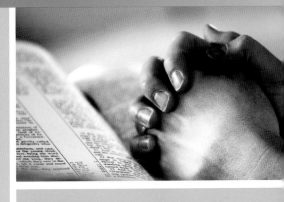

»Medical

If you forget to take your medication for one dose, do not take a double dose. Instead, call your primary care provider and ask whether you should take a dose immediately, or wait until it is time for the next dose to get back on track.

»Movement

Today work out your arms while you get some cardio exercise. Go for a walk and carry some light hand-weights (two or five pounds—nothing heavier). Do some bicep curls as you walk.

{ The fruit of wellness is life. }

» Work

How has this journey impacted your work life thus far? Have you noticed changes in your attitude, your work ethic, your productivity? Consider how you have changed your work life today and take note of your improvements.

» Emotional

Take ten minutes and check in with your current emotional state. Do you feel good? Discouraged? Frustrated? Write about what you are feeling, particularly in relation to your wellness journey.

» Family and Friends

Today go out to a favorite restaurant with some friends or family. Again, try to enjoy the company and the socializing more than the food. Enjoy the food, but make the social interaction the star of the evening.

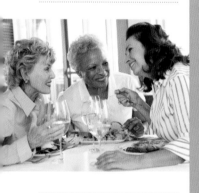

» Nutrition

Do not eat at the first sign of hunger. Instead, wait until you are feeling strong feelings of hunger to eat, because when you start to get hungry your body taps into your fat stores for energy.

Evening Wrap-Up

Up to this point, our weight-management journey has been full of ups and downs and ins and outs. But as we move forward, it is important to remember that we walk this journey with small steps. We take these small steps toward weight management and wellness because we are making lifestyle changes. In the Gospel of Luke, Jesus tells us not to worry. We are assured that God walks with us on the journey. It is not for us to worry but to continue on the journey.

> Then Jesus said to his disciples: "Therefore I tell you, do not worry about your life, what you will eat; or about your body, what you will wear. For life is more than food, and the body more than clothes. Consider the ravens: They do not sow or reap, they have no storeroom or barn; yet God feeds them."
>
> LUKE 12:22–24

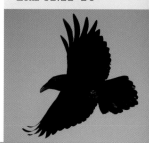

Loving God, help me today to focus on the path ahead of me on my journey to weight management. In Your holy name, Amen.

Morning Reflection

Today is day thirty-five, the final day of week five.
We are coming to the end of our six-week journey, but really we are coming to the beginning of the larger journey—living life. Consider Jesus' forty days in the wilderness. It was preparation for the rest of His life. Those forty days were not His entire life. Our six-week journey is preparation for the weight-management journey that will come after we have completed six weeks.

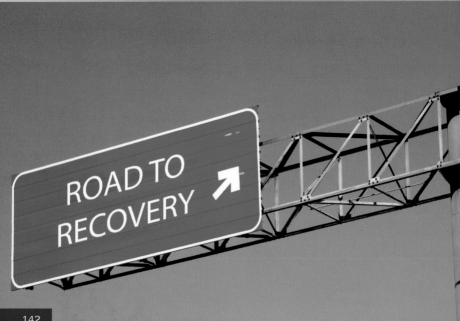

»Faith Life

Today read Luke 8:40–56.
Then spend five minutes
writing about when you
have experienced God's
healing grace in your life.
Keep in mind God heals in
many different ways.

....

....

....

....

....

....

....

....

....

{ Your six-week
journey is the
preparation for
the wellness
journey after the
six weeks are
completed. }

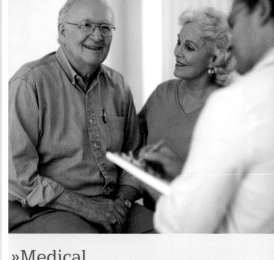

»Medical

**By this point on the journey, we hope that
you will be seeing and feeling some difference in your body.** If you are not feeling
or looking different, take heart! Everyone's
progress is different, but you may also want to
speak with your doctor about how your weight
management is progressing.

»Movement

Exercise is incredibly healing. Today spend
ten minutes warming up your muscles with
some jumping jacks or jogging in place. Then
spend at least five minutes stretching your
muscles.

....

143

»Work

Today at work, if you are stuck sitting for long periods of time, try to move your feet by bouncing your legs up and down, or even rolling your ankles around. This will help maintain circulation in your legs and can help relieve pain or swelling that comes with that much sitting.

»Emotional

Physical healing means very little without emotional healing. Take ten minutes and write about a time in your life that you experienced emotional healing, such as a time when you have forgiven or been forgiven.

»Family and Friends

A large part of any healing is our support system. Today have a conversation with the members of your family and friends who are an important part of your support system. Tell them what healing on this journey looks like for you.

»Nutrition

Cheese is one of the main sources of saturated fat. Today switch to a 2 percent milk cheese and pay attention to portion size. (One serving of cheese is an ounce, about the size of six dice.)

Evening Wrap-Up

We are all children of God, or as this passage from Acts says, "We are His offspring." God walks this journey with us and will continue the journey with us well past the six-week mark, and God will offer us healing. This journey is one of physical healing in many ways, but also a journey of spiritual healing. Today as we look back on the weeks, we can celebrate and give thanks for the healing that God has given us.

"From one man he made all the nations, that they should inhabit the whole earth. . . . God did this so that they would seek him and perhaps reach out for him and find him, though he is not far from any one of us. 'For in him we live and move and have our being.' As some of your own poets have said, 'We are his offspring.'"

ACTS 17:26–28

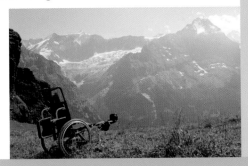

Loving God, help my body and my spirit to heal as I continue on my journey to wellness. In Your holy name, Amen.

Six years ago Lawrence was living in Louisiana.

Like many other members of his family, Lawrence suffered from diabetes, asthma, and other complications from his weight. His mother Corinne was in a similar physical situation before suddenly passing away. On the day that she died, Lawrence had a dream where his mother appeared to him and told him not to go the way she had. After that dream, he knew that he needed to make changes to lose weight, but he didn't know how to address the immense work he had in front of him.

Soon after her death, Hurricane Katrina swept away his community, and Lawrence and his family came to Memphis. He was still grieving the death of his mother, devastated by the disaster in Louisiana, and challenged by his weight problems. He became depressed and was losing hope when he learned about the Church Health Center. Suddenly, he remembered the promise he had made to his mother and showed up at the Wellness Center with a spirit of determination.

Lawrence and his whole family have now become members of the center and have collectively lost almost a thousand pounds! He still misses his home in Louisiana—and misses his mother most of all—but he and his family have found a new community of friends at the Church Health Center.

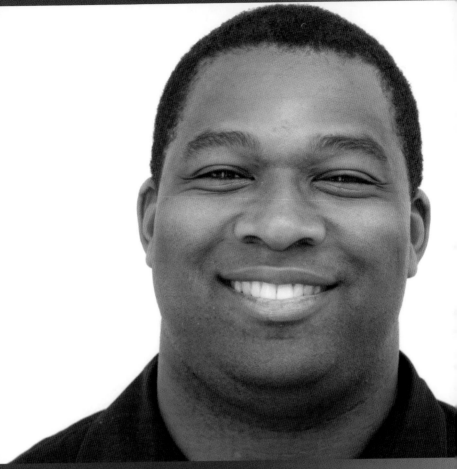

Suddenly, he remembered the promise he had made to his mother and showed up at the Wellness Center with a spirit of determination.

Weight Management

Morning Reflection

Congratulations! We have reached the final days

of this six-week journey toward weight management. We now have a story of our journey. It is the story of a conversion and a changing life. As we know, some conversions happen quickly and others happen slowly over time. For most of us, our conversion stories are a combination of a sudden conversion paired with a longer journey. We may have a moment when we realize that we need to change our lives. But it is only in the longer journey that we are actually changed.

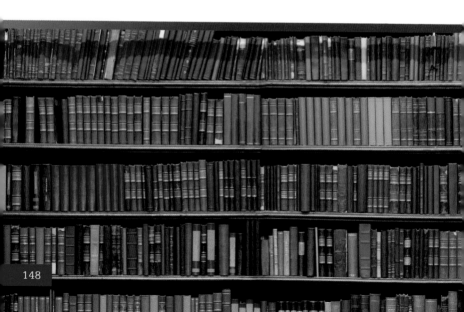

»Faith Life

Today try a walking meditation. Go for a slow walk around your neighborhood without a specific plan. Simply let yourself wander for about ten minutes. Try to quiet yourself and just walk.

{ It is only in the longer journey that we are actually changed. }

»Medical

The next time you have a doctor's appointment, discuss the lifestyle changes that you have made over the last six weeks with your doctor. Your doctor may have some insight into ways that you can make further progress from here.

»Movement

Getting regular exercise can lower your risk of diseases such as diabetes, heart disease, and arthritis. Today go for a walk and try to raise your heart rate. Make sure that you breathe deeply as your heart rate rises.

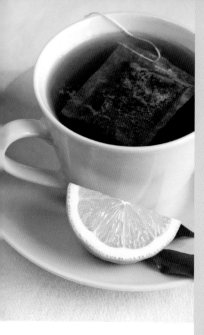

»Work

Bring a stash of non-caffeinated, non-sweetened herbal teas into work. When you feel like drinking a cup of coffee, have a cup of herbal tea instead. That way you will be more hydrated and you will avoid the bursts of energy and crashes that come with caffeine and sugar.

»Emotional

Many times, quick conversions are what we could call mountaintop experiences. But the real work is done in the valleys. Today write about times that you have been on the mountaintop and how those experiences translate to the work in the valleys.

»Family and Friends

Often, our family and friends are not on exactly the same path to conversion as we are. Today if your family and friends do not seem to understand why you are on the journey, tell them your conversion story to help them understand where you are coming from.

»Nutrition

If you eat canned fruit instead of fresh fruit, rinse the fruit off before you eat it. This will wash away some of the excess sugar and syrup that the fruit comes in. (Hint: frozen fruit is often available and contains less excess sugar than canned.)

Evening Wrap-Up

We all know the story of Saul's conversion on the road to Damascus.

He got knocked off a horse, changed his name, and the rest is history, right? Except that after he fell off his horse, Paul still had a long road ahead of him in the days and weeks and years after the road to Damascus. Likewise, our journey to wellness does not stop at the end of these six weeks. Instead, the real journey is the long road ahead of us: life.

As he neared Damascus on his journey, suddenly a light from heaven flashed around him. He fell to the ground and heard a voice say to him, "Saul, Saul, why do you persecute me?" "Who are you, Lord?" Saul asked. "I am Jesus, whom you are persecuting," he replied. "Now get up and go into the city, and you will be told what you must do."

ACTS 9:3–6

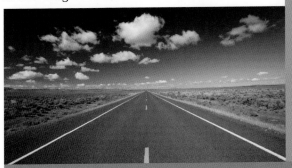

Loving God, help me on the journey ahead of me to embrace the small steps. In Your holy name, Amen.

Morning Reflection

This journey to weight management has never been just about numbers on a scale. The journey has been about learning how to live a new life and about learning to live the life that we have been given to its fullest potential. The journey to weight management and wellness generally is about learning to see and care for ourselves in the same way that God sees and cares for us. So today we will turn our focus to how we can embrace this life that we have been given.

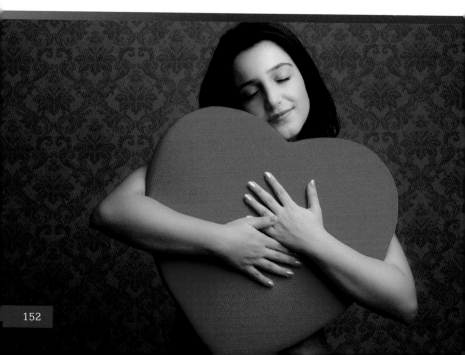

»Faith Life

The first step in "Love your neighbor as yourself" is to love yourself. Today spend five minutes writing about what it means to love yourself. Remember that God loves you.

....

....

....

....

....

....

....

....

....

....

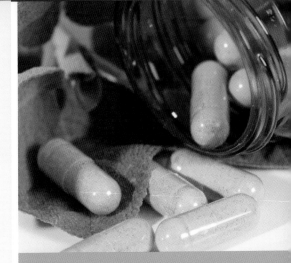

{ Today we will try to see ourselves as God sees us. }

»Medical

Before you start taking a vitamin or supplement, consult your health care provider. Sometimes vitamins and supplements can have interactions with prescription medications that would not be listed on the bottle.

....

....

»Movement

Today spend ten minutes stretching and exploring all of the parts that God made. Touch your toes, cross your arms over your chest, roll your neck, stretch your arms up over your head, and stretch your back.

....

153

» Work

If you must go out for lunch at work, try to avoid eating fast food. Instead, try to find a place where you can order lean protein and vegetables that are not fried.

» Emotional

One of the keys to emotional wellness is to spend time engaged in self-care. Today write down one area in your life where you could use some more self-care. Do you need to find some extra alone time? Do you need to schedule more time with friends?

» Family and Friends

When you plan activities with your family and friends, try going to a park, playground, or museum instead of going immediately to a restaurant. This way you will have some kind of physical activity built into your outing.

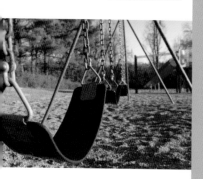

» Nutrition

Know exactly what you are eating. When you go shopping, make sure to read the food label before you buy the food. The ingredients listed first are the major ingredients in that product.

Evening Wrap-Up

Jesus tells us that He came so that we would have life, and life

in abundance. But what does that mean for us? As we end this six-week journey, we have worked on making some significant and not-so-significant changes in our day-to-day lives. Those changes, we hope, will help us to live our lives more fully.

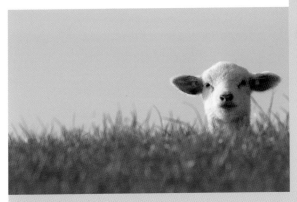

Therefore Jesus said again, "Very truly I tell you, I am the gate for the sheep. All who have come before me are thieves and robbers, but the sheep have not listened to them. I am the gate; whoever enters through me will be saved. They will come in and go out, and find pasture. The thief comes only to steal and kill and destroy; I have come that they may have life, and have it to the full."

JOHN 10:7–10

God of abundant love, help me today and all days to see myself as You see me, and to care for myself as You care for all creation. In Your holy name, Amen.

Morning Reflection

Our days on this six-week journey are very limited at this point. As we look forward, we need to be setting up our support for the journey yet to come. After all, this weight-management journey is a lifelong journey. It is not a goal that can be attained and then left behind. Throughout the journey to this point, we have been working to put habits and lifestyle changes into place to prepare us for the next steps. Today we will consider what those next steps will be.

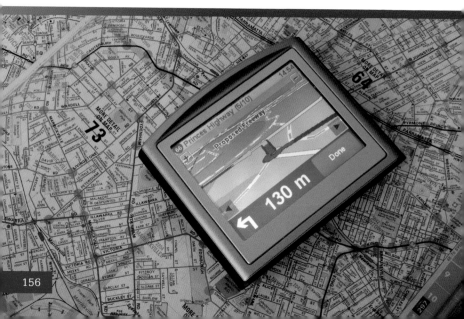

» Faith Life

Our faith can be an anchor for us when things become challenging. Today spend five minutes writing about the things, people, places, and activities that give you hope on your journey.

» Medical

If you find yourself beginning to engage in obsessive behaviors when it comes to food and exercise, make sure that you speak to your doctor about it.

» Movement

If you run to the store to buy a gallon of milk, carry the milk with you instead of putting it in a cart. Then while you stand in line, do some alternating bicep curls with it.

» Work

Bring an insulated lunch bag to work with some raw chopped vegetables such as celery, carrots, and red bell peppers to snack on when you get hungry. If you want to add a little spice, throw in a few radishes as well.

» Emotional

Branching out into the next part of the journey can be intimidating. Today make a list of activities that help you relieve your stress.

» Family and Friends

Your family and friends will be very important to your journey. Today try to set up a regular walking time with (at least) one of your friends or family members. Having a regular time will help you to get into (and stay in) the habit of walking.

» Nutrition

If you are tired of eating so many servings of vegetables each day (aim for five), try swapping out one serving of raw or cooked vegetables with a half cup of vegetable juice. Be sure to account for added sugar in the juice!

But you, dear friends, by building yourselves up in your most holy faith and praying in the Holy Spirit, keep yourselves in God's love as you wait for the mercy of our Lord Jesus Christ to bring you to eternal life.

JUDE 20–21

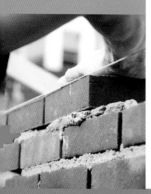

Evening Wrap-Up

As we bring this journey to a close,

we should keep in mind that the journey forward is about hope. God offers us that hope as we move forward. We have skills and knowledge necessary to be healthy and to continue the journey. But what will keep us on the journey is the support that comes from God's love and from the love and support of those around us. As Jude reminds us, "build yourselves up." As we move forward, it is important to work on those practices and habits that will continue to build ourselves up.

Loving God, help me today as I begin to look down the road. Grant me hope and encouragement for what is to come. In Your holy name, Amen.

Morning Reflection

We are approaching the final stretch of this six-week journey, and we need to be reminded that we are not alone on the journey. Though it is true that we are, in most cases, trying to change individual habits, the people who surround us can give us encouragement. Think of Lawrence and his family! They got healthy together, encouraging one another and making life changes as a family. Today we will focus on ways that we can surround ourselves with fellow travelers on the journey.

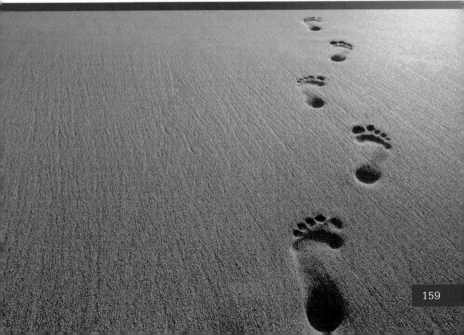

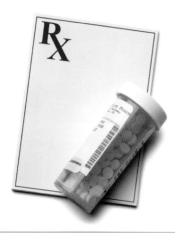

»Faith Life

Does your faith community have Sunday school programs? Today consider starting up a Sunday school program that is centered on the wellness journey. Encourage other members of your faith community to live wellness-oriented lives.

»Medical

Remember that medication is not a magical pill. When your physician writes a prescription for a medication, ask questions about what lifestyle changes you should be making along with the medication to be healthier.

»Movement

Today before you eat dinner, do some cardio exercise. Go for a walk, or jog in place for five minutes, or do thirty jumping jacks. Exercising before eating will make you healthier, and will in turn motivate you to eat healthier.

> We need to be reminded that we are not alone on the journey.

»Work

If there is someone at your work who shares your particular lunchtime and perhaps is interested in eating healthy meals, adopt that person as a lunch buddy. Take turns bringing in new, healthy dishes to try.

»Emotional

When we feel alone, we can become despondent, and it can really halt our progress on the wellness journey. Today spend five minutes writing about the many ways in which you are not alone.

»Family and Friends

Your family and friends can be of great support, but it can also be good to seek support from people who are going through a very similar experience to you. Support groups exist at gyms and wellness centers as well as online. Find a group that you can belong to.

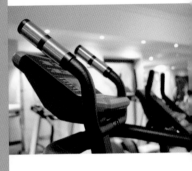

»Nutrition

No matter how much you want to lose weight, do not start a fad diet. While they may help you lose weight, fad diets generally do not promote overall wellness. You will be better off with long-term lifestyle changes.

Evening Wrap-Up

I always thank my God as I remember you in my prayers, because I hear about your love for all his holy people and your faith in the Lord Jesus. I pray that your partnership with us in the faith may be effective in deepening your understanding of every good thing we share for the sake of Christ. Your love has given me great joy and encouragement, because you, brother, have refreshed the hearts of the Lord's people.

PHILEMON 4—7

Many of us look to Paul as an ultimate example of discipleship and devotion to Christ. But Paul did not do it alone. Paul took a great deal of encouragement from people in his life. We are all called to live in community, to support one another, and to encourage one another. On this journey to weight management, we can rest assured that we are loved and supported, and we can take encouragement from that.

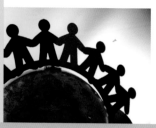

Loving God, thank You for loving me. Give me strength to continue on this journey and to encourage others who are also on the journey. In Your holy name, Amen.

Morning Reflection

Today is day forty—congratulations! You have made it forty days! Over the past six weeks you have gained the skills necessary to continue on your journey toward weight management. Setbacks will probably happen from time to time, but in the last six weeks, you have set up a foundation that you can return to when needed. The journey to wellness may take you to unexpected places, but wherever wellness takes you, it is sure to lead to a fuller and more abundant life.

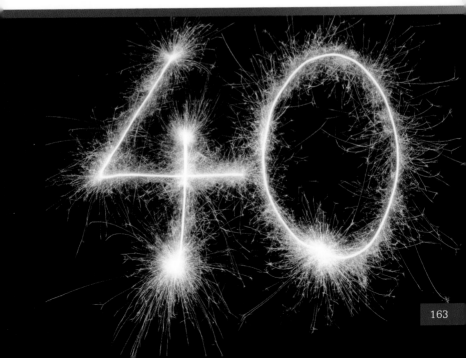

» Faith Life

What does "abundant life" mean to you? We are told that Jesus came so that we might have life, and life in abundance. What might that mean for you?

» Medical

If you change health care providers, try to get to know them while you are healthy. It is much easier for doctors to treat you when they know what the "healthy you" is like.

» Movement

In celebration of life in abundance, put on some music and dance today. Bounce around, get your heart rate up, and don't forget to use your arms!

» Work

If you need to go out to lunch for work, ask for a "to-go" box to come out with your food. If the portions are larger than what is healthy (as is the case at most restaurants) put half of your order in the box before you eat.

» Emotional

Today try to rest. When we are tired, overworked, and sleep deprived, our body responds to stressors, causing us to hang on to weight and generally feel icky. Even if you only manage to take a twenty-minute nap, it will help you feel better.

» Family and Friends

Today prepare a meal for your friends and family that you have never prepared before. Get your guests to help you prepare the meal, chopping vegetables or stirring the pot as things cook.

» Nutrition

Do not skip breakfast! If you want a change from the usual cereal, try eating leftovers from last night's dinner for breakfast. That will get you at least a serving of vegetables to start out the day.

Evening Wrap-Up

Remember that God gives us abundant grace through Jesus Christ and that we are not only given abundant grace in spirit, but in our whole selves and our whole lives. This journey to wellness is about responding appropriately to that abundant grace that Jesus Christ grants us. When we care for ourselves, we are caring for God's creation—the very thing that Jesus came to save.

For if, by the trespass of the one man, death reigned through that one man, how much more will those who receive God's abundant provision of grace and of the gift of righteousness reign in life through the one man, Jesus Christ!

ROMANS 5:17

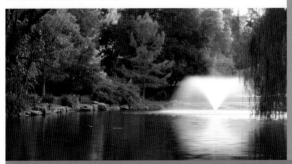

Gracious Lord, thank You for walking with me on this journey and for the abundant grace that You give me. Help me today and all days to live my life to abundance in wellness and in grace. In Your holy name, Amen.

Morning Reflection

Now that the forty days are over, today will be a day of review. When we started out on this journey, we had to assess where we were in order to set goals for the road ahead. In a similar manner, we have to assess where we are again, so that we can know where we need to go from here. We need to see our successes as well as our setbacks, so that we know what we still need to work on.

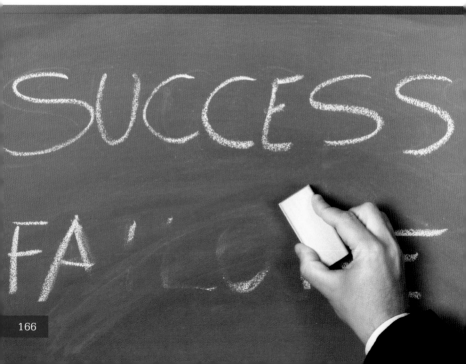

»Faith Life

When we started, you wrote ten words describing your faith life. Again, take five minutes and write ten words describing your faith life now. Then compare the two lists. What has changed? What has stayed the same?

....

....

....

....

....

....

....

....

....

»Medical

What are your medical concerns now? Are they significantly different from what they were six weeks ago? Write down your current medical concerns, but do not get rid of your old list of concerns.

....

....

....

....

»Movement

Go for a walk today, and walk as far as you can walk. How far could you walk the first time you did this? Can you feel the improvement in the way your body is reacting to the walking?

....

....

....

....

{ We need to see our successes as well as our setbacks. }

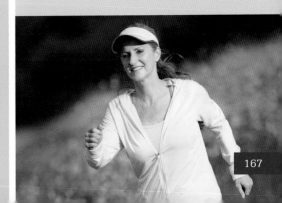

» Work

What has changed about your work environment? Are you drinking more water? Are you eating healthier snacks? Are you getting a little exercise throughout the day?

» Emotional

What has changed in your emotional wellness? Take a look at your emotional highs and lows from week two. Do you still have similar highs and lows, or has your overall emotional pattern changed a bit?

» Family and Friends

What have your family and friends thought about your journey? Can they see a difference in you? Take a moment today and ask one or two of them.

» Nutrition

In the first week, you made a list of the foods that you like to eat. Can you expand that list any after six weeks? In particular, can you include more healthy meals on that list?

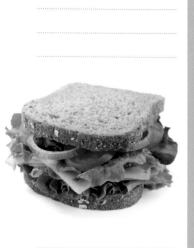

Evening Wrap-Up

The last six weeks have been challenging in a variety of ways.

You have been asked to try vastly new things, from food to exercises. You have been asked to step outside of your comfort zone and explore emotions that most of us do not take the time to explore regularly. But the journey—at least this part of the journey—is finished. And you have finished the race. For that, you ought to be very proud and thankful. You have run the race, and God has been running right beside you. Remember as you continue from this point, God runs the race with you. God gives us all strength and endurance when we most need it, and God cheers when we cross the finish line.

I have fought the good fight, I have finished the race, I have kept the faith. . . . But the Lord stood at my side and gave me strength. . . . To him be glory for ever and ever. Amen.

2 TIMOTHY 4:7, 17–18

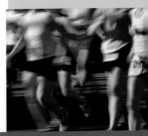

God of strength, thank You for the gift of wellness. Help me to continue on this journey with endurance and bravery. In Your holy name, Amen.

Morning Reflection

With the six weeks completed, it can certainly feel like the journey is over. However, as we have said before, the journey has really only just begun. The journey to wellness is never over. Life will offer us many surprises along the way, and it will be part of the journey to adapt as life happens. Today as we close this chapter on the journey, we look ahead to continue the lessons learned on this journey.

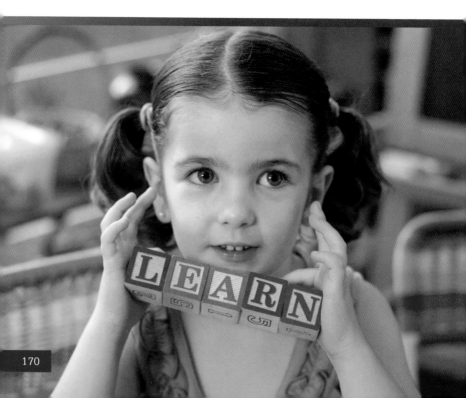

»Faith Life

As you continue on this journey, remember to take time to pray or meditate each day. Prayer and meditation can keep you connected to your purpose and your anchor.

»Medical

Take all medication exactly as prescribed, and do not be afraid to talk to your doctor about anything. The best way to stay medically healthy is to have open communication with your doctor and other health care providers.

»Movement

Move everywhere. Find ways to add a few steps to your day in everything that you do. A great goal would be to add two hundred steps the first day, then three hundred, then four hundred, and to keep adding up as much as you can. That will help your body to burn calories more efficiently each day.

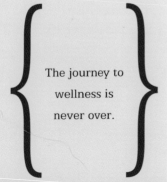

{ The journey to wellness is never over. }

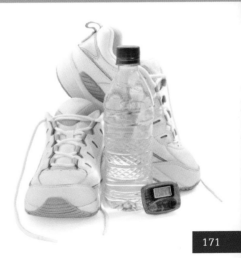

»Work

Try to find time in your days to exercise even a little bit. It will help break up the monotony of the day, and will help you to add a few steps.

»Emotional

Find and remember ways that you can relieve stress. Take a hot bath, go for a walk, or read a book. Just find something that works for you and do it every day. The more you relieve your stress, the better you will feel, and the healthier you will become.

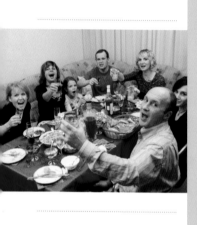

»Family and Friends

Remember that your family and friends are your support system. When you are struggling, do not be afraid to lean on them for support, and when you have succeeded, do not be afraid to celebrate with them.

»Nutrition

Make your calories count. Enjoy all the wonderful colors and flavors of God's creation as you prepare meals using whole grains, a variety of fruits and vegetables, and lean meats—but let yourself splurge on occasion!

Evening Wrap-Up

It has been a long journey to this point, but you have been given many tools to continue. You will find other tools to add to your toolbox, and you will have setbacks. But remember that God walks with you, and God can grant you peace, even when you have a difficult time finding it for yourself.

Finally, brothers and sisters, whatever is true, whatever is noble, whatever is right, whatever is pure, whatever is lovely, whatever is admirable—if anything is excellent or praiseworthy—think about such things. Whatever you have learned or received or heard from me, or seen in me—put it into practice. And the God of peace will be with you.

PHILIPPIANS 4:8–9

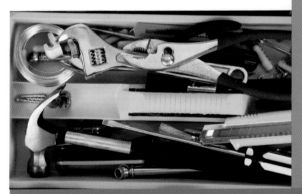

Sustaining Lord, be with me as I continue on this journey. Help me to remember the things I have learned, and help me to continue learning. I will continue to strive to honor my body and my whole self, Your creation. In Your holy name, Amen.

Recommended Reading and Resources

Websites

Church Health Reader, www.chreader.org. Church Health Reader is the online and print publication of the Church Health Center. Church Health Reader provides resources for you and your church to become healthier in body and spirit. It offers interviews with leaders and thinkers, tips and advice on running effective ministries, and practical suggestions for individuals and churches. The print version is published four times a year and is available through yearly subscription or online at www.chreader.org.

Books

Regaining the Power of Youth at Any Age by Kenneth H. Cooper. This book features a scientifically based program that will guide you to a higher level of physical and mental fitness that you may have believed impossible to attain.

What to Eat by Marion Nestle. Nestle walks readers through every supermarket section—produce, meat, fish, dairy, packaged foods, bottled waters, and more—decoding labels and clarifying nutritional and other claims (in supermarket-speak, for example, "fresh" means most likely to spoil first, not recently picked or prepared), and in so doing explores issues like the effects of food production on our environment, the way pricing works, and additives and their effect on nutrition.

The Inner Game of Stress: Outsmart Life's Challenges and Fulfill Your Potential by W. Timothy Gallwey. Renowned sports psychology expert W. Timothy Gallwey teams up with two esteemed physicians to offer a unique and empowering guide to mental health in today's volatile world. *The Inner Game of Stress* applies the trusted principles of Gallwey's wildly popular Inner Game series, which have helped athletes the world over, to the management of everyday stress— personal, professional, financial, physical—and shows us how to access our inner resources to maintain stability and achieve success.

Your Child's Weight: Helping without Harming by Ellyn Satter. As much about parenting as feeding, this latest release from renowned childhood feeding expert Ellyn Satter considers the overweight child issue in a new way. Combining scientific research with inspiring anecdotes from her decades of clinical practice, Satter challenges the conventional belief that parents must get overweight children to eat less and exercise more.

Mindless Eating: Why We Eat More Than We Think by Brian Wansink. In this illuminating and groundbreaking new book, food psychologist Brian Wansink shows why you may not realize how much you're eating, what you're eating—or why you're even eating at all.

Change or Die: The Three Keys to Change at Work and in Life by Alan Deutschman. A powerful book with universal appeal, *Change or Die* deconstructs and debunks age-old myths about change and empowers us with three critical keys—relate, repeat, and reframe—to help us make important positive changes in our lives. Explaining breakthrough research and progressive ideas from a wide selection of leaders in medicine, science, and business, Deutschman demonstrates how anyone can achieve lasting, revolutionary changes that are positive, attainable, and absolutely vital.

Family Health, Nutrition and Fitness by Paul C. Reisser. This book will help you take an active role in improving the health and well-being of you and your family by offering authoritative and current medical information in a convenient, easy-to-understand format. Taking a balanced, commonsense approach to the issue of health and wellness, this indispensable guide delivers an encouraging perspective with helpful reference sections.

40 Days to Better Living

A series of practical books
dealing with specific health issues

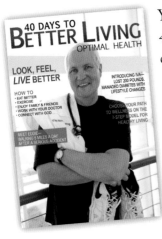

You want to feel better—and *40 Days to Better Living* provides clear, manageable steps to get you there through life-changing attitudes and actions. If you're ready to live better, select one or more elements of the Seven-Step Model for Healthy Living—Faith Life, Medical, Movement, Work, Emotional, Family and Friends, and Nutrition—and follow the forty-day plan to improve your life, just a bit, day-by-day. With plenty of practical advice, biblical encouragement, and stories of real people who have taken the same journey, this may be the most important book you read this year!

Bimonthly release schedule, through 2013.

Titles to include:

Optimal Health / Hypertension / Depression /
Rest & Relaxation / Weight Management /
Stress Management / Aging / Addiction /
Diabetes / Anxiety / Caregiving